Pediatrics:

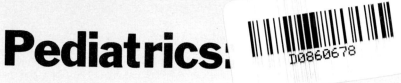

PreTest® Self-Assessment and Review

Fourth Edition

Edited by

Richard E. Kravath, M.D., F.A.A.P.
Professor of Clinical Pediatrics
State University of New York, Health Science Center at Brooklyn,
  College of Medicine
New York, New York

Director, In-Patient Pediatric Service
Kings County Hospital Center
New York, New York

McGraw-Hill Book Company
Health Professions Division
PreTest Series

New York St. Louis San Francisco
Auckland Bogotá Hamburg
Lisbon London Madrid Mexico
Milan Montreal New Delhi Panama
Paris San Juan São Paulo Singapore
Sydney Tokyo Toronto

Notice

Medicine is an ever-changing science. As new research and clinical experience broaden our knowledge, changes in treatment and drug therapy are required. The editor and the publisher of this work have checked with sources believed to be reliable in their efforts to provide drug dosage schedules that are complete and in accord with the standards accepted at the time of publication. However, readers are advised to check the product information sheet included in the package of each drug they plan to administer to be certain that the information contained in these schedules is accurate and that changes have not been made in the recommended dose or in the contraindications for administration. This recommendation is of particular importance in connection with new or infrequently used drugs.

Library of Congress Cataloging-in-Publication Data

Pediatrics: PreTest self-assessment and review.

Bibliography: p.
1. Pediatrics—Examinations, questions, etc.
I. Kravath, Richard E. [DNLM: 1. Pediatrics—
examination questions. WS 18 P371]
RJ48.2.P42   1987   618.92'00076   86-33781
ISBN 0-07-051015-6

This book was set in English Times (Times Roman) by Waldman Graphics, Inc.; the editors were Eileen J. Scott and Bruce MacGregor; the production supervisor was Clara B. Stanley.
Semline, Inc., was printer and binder.

2 3 4 5 6 7 8 9 0   SEMSEM   8 9 4 3 2 1 0 9 8 7

ISBN 0-07-051015-6

Contents

Introduction

Pediatrics: PreTest Self-Assessment and Review, 4th Ed. provides comprehensive self-assessment and review within the field of pediatrics. The 500 questions contained in the book have been designed to be similar in format and degree of difficulty to the questions contained in the Part II examination of the National Board of Medical Examiners, the Federation Licensing Examination (FLEX), and the Foreign Medical Graduate Examination in the Medical Sciences (FMGEMS).

Each question has the correct answer, an explanation, and a specific reference to either a current journal article, a textbook, or both. A bibliography, listing the sources used in the book, follows the last chapter.

Perhaps the most effective way to use this book is to allow yourself about one minute to answer each question in a given chapter in order to approximate the time limits imposed by the examinations previously mentioned. As you proceed, indicate your answer to each question.

When you have finished answering the questions in a chapter, you should then spend as much time as you need verifying your answers and reading the explanations. Although you should pay special attention to the explanations for the questions you answered incorrectly, you should read every explanation. The author has designed the explanations to reinforce and supplement the information tested by the questions. If, after reading the explanations you want more information, you should consult and study the references indicated.

This book meets the criteria for up to 22 credit hours in Category 5(D) for the Physician's Recognition Award of the American Medical Association. We hope it provides an experience that is instructive as well as evaluative; we also hope that you enjoy it. We would be happy to receive your comments.

General Pediatrics

DIRECTIONS: Each question below contains five suggested responses. Select the **one best** response to each question.

1. Estimation of the surface area of a burn requires knowledge of how the body's total surface area is apportioned. The chief difference between infants and adults is that infants have a proportionally

(A) smaller surface area for the trunk
(B) smaller surface area for the genitals
(C) smaller surface area for the hands and feet
(D) larger surface area for the head and neck
(E) larger surface area for the buttocks

2. The vector of typhus, trench fever, and relapsing fever is

(A) *Pediculus humanis capitis*
(B) *Pediculus humanis pedis*
(C) *Pediculus humanis corporis*
(D) *Phthirius pubis*
(E) *Dermacentor andersoni*

3. Sudden infant death syndrome has all the following characteristics EXCEPT that

(A) it affects female infants predominantly
(B) it typically involves infants 2 to 4 months of age
(C) it is more common among siblings of affected infants
(D) it has a higher incidence among infants of drug-addicted mothers
(E) it has a higher incidence among infants of lower socioeconomic status

4. Salicylate poisoning is most likely to be associated with which of the following?

(A) Respiratory acidosis followed by metabolic alkalosis
(B) Respiratory alkalosis followed by metabolic alkalosis
(C) Respiratory alkalosis followed by metabolic acidosis
(D) Metabolic acidosis superimposed upon respiratory alkalosis
(E) Metabolic acidosis superimposed upon respiratory acidosis

1

5. All the following are manifestations of chronic hypervitaminosis A EXCEPT for

(A) hepatomegaly
(B) alopecia
(C) desquamation of palms and soles
(D) tender swelling of bones
(E) subcutaneous calcifications

6. Iridocyclitis (anterior uveitis), which is depicted in the photograph below, is most likely to be associated with which of the following disorders?

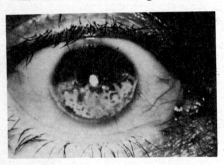

(A) Juvenile rheumatoid arthritis
(B) Slipped femoral epiphysis
(C) Schönlein-Henoch purpura
(D) Legg-Calvé-Perthes disease
(E) Osgood-Schlatter disease

7. Lyme arthritis is usually preceded by a characteristic rash that is

(A) erythema marginatum
(B) erythema multiforme
(C) erythema chronicum migrans
(D) urticaria
(E) morbilliform

8. A buccal smear is performed on a child to determine the presence and number of Barr bodies; the nucleus of a buccal cell is shown below. The sex-chromosome pattern of this cell is

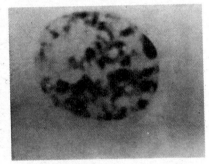

(A) XO
(B) XY
(C) XX
(D) XXX
(E) XXXX

9. The child shown below was brought to the emergency room because of an inability to urinate. The most likely diagnosis is

(A) priapism
(B) balanitis
(C) balanoposthitis
(D) phimosis
(E) paraphimosis

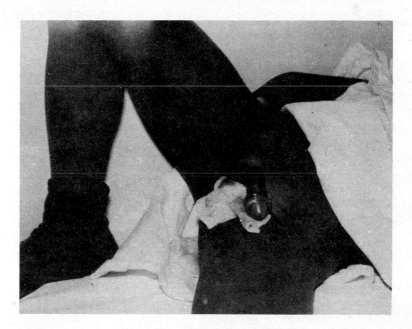

10. In children, the most commonly recognized form of familial hyperlipidemia is

(A) hypertriglyceridemia
(B) hypercholesterolemia
(C) hyperchylomicronemia
(D) combined hyperlipidemia
(E) type V hyperlipoproteinemia

11. Osgood-Schlatter disease involves the

(A) tarsal navicular
(B) metatarsal head
(C) capital femoral epiphysis
(D) tibial tuberosity
(E) body of the sternum

12. The International Code of Ethics for Biomedical Research includes all the following principles EXCEPT

(A) biomedical research involving human subjects must conform to generally accepted scientific principles and should be based on adequately performed laboratory and animal experimentation and thorough knowledge of the scientific literature

(B) the design and performance of each experimental procedure involving human subjects should be clearly formulated in an experimental protocol, which should be transmitted to a specially appointed independent committee for consideration, comment, and guidance

(C) biomedical research involving human subjects should be conducted only by scientifically qualified persons and under the supervision of a clinically competent medical person. The responsibility for the human subject must always rest with a medically qualified person and never rest with the subject of the research, even though the subject has given his or her consent

(D) biomedical research involving human subjects cannot legitimately be done unless the importance of the objective is in proportion to the inherent risk to the subject

(E) each potential subject should be informed that he or she is at liberty to abstain from participation in the study and may withdraw consent for participation at any time until the actual experiment has started

13. The results in a study of a new treatment favored the new treatment (P $\langle$.05). This means that

(A) the new treatment is 5 percent better than the old treatment

(B) a critical threshold for medical significance has been reached

(C) five percent of the time patients will not benefit from the new therapy

(D) the odds are less than one in twenty that the differences observed were only a chance variation

(E) it would be unethical to continue the old treatment

14. The two formulations of a drug that have been found to be of equal value by clinical trial may be said to be

(A) therapeutically equivalent

(B) biologically equivalent

(C) chemically equivalent

(D) different in bioavailability

(E) identical

15. A 6-year-old asthmatic child is brought to the emergency room because of severe coughing and wheezing during the prior 24 hours. The child had been taking theophylline without relief. Physical examination reveals a child who is anxious, has intercostal and suprasternal retractions, expiratory wheezing throughout all lung fields, and a respiratory rate of 60 per minute. Initial treatment may include the administration of

(A) intravenous penicillin
(B) parenteral phenobarbital
(C) subcutaneous epinephrine
(D) enough intravenous fluids in the first 2 hours to correct a deficit of 100 ml/kg
(E) N-acetyl cysteine and cromolyn by inhaler

16. Pityriasis rosea is a common, benign rash in children, characterized by a herald patch that usually precedes the generalized eruption. The etiologic agent of the disease is

(A) viral
(B) mycobacterial
(C) fungal
(D) spirochetal
(E) unknown

17. Evaluation of cerebrospinal fluid is critical in evaluating children of all ages for possible central nervous system infections. Normally, the CSF should contain no more than five leukocytes and the protein should be 10–30 mg/dl. However, in newborns the values are different. Which of the following combinations is most typical?

(A) Up to 15 leukocytes, 5,000 red cells, and 300 mg/dl protein
(B) Up to 5 leukocytes and less than 10 mg/dl protein
(C) Up to 15 leukocytes, 500 red cells, and 100 mg/dl protein
(D) Zero cells and 100 mg/dl protein
(E) Up to 100 red blood cells and 300 mg/dl protein

18. Treatment of a child who has acute lead encephalopathy should include prompt administration of

(A) edetate calcium disodium (Ca EDTA)
(B) edetate calcium disodium and dimercaprol (British anti-lewisite)
(C) D-penicillamine
(D) D-penicillamine and dimercaprol
(E) D-penicillamine, edetate calcium disodium, and dimercaprol

Questions 19–20

An 8-month-old girl is admitted to a hospital because of poor weight gain despite a voracious appetite. The presence of steatorrhea and a right upper lobe pneumonia points to cystic fibrosis.

19. If cystic fibrosis is the correct diagnosis, results of her sweat test would be expected to show

(A) low sodium and chloride concentrations
(B) low sodium concentration and high chloride concentration
(C) normal sodium and chloride concentrations
(D) high sodium concentration and normal chloride concentration
(E) high sodium and chloride concentrations

20. The parents of the girl described want to know whether future offspring also will be born with cystic fibrosis. They should be advised that the chance that their next child will have the disease is approximately

(A) 0 percent
(B) 25 percent
(C) 33 percent
(D) 50 percent
(E) 100 percent

21. The child pictured below has the most common type of generalized skeletal dysplasia. The disorder is

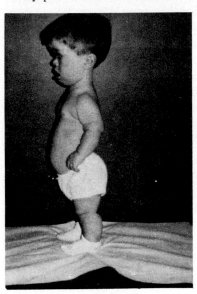

(A) achondrogenesis
(B) achondroplasia
(C) metatropic dwarfism
(D) thanatophoric dwarfism
(E) chondroectodermal dysplasia

22. The bone most frequently fractured at the time of delivery is the

(A) cranium
(B) radius
(C) femur
(D) tibia
(E) clavicle

23. Milk is indicated after ingestion of a poison

(A) to distend the stomach after giving ipecac
(B) when a caustic agent has been ingested and prompt endoscopy is not planned
(C) as a dilutant for activated charcoal
(D) following irritant ingestions prior to endoscopy
(E) in place of activated charcoal for amphetamine poisoning

DIRECTIONS: Each question below contains four suggested responses of which **one or more** is correct. Select

A	if	**1, 2, and 3**	are correct
B	if	**1 and 3**	are correct
C	if	**2 and 4**	are correct
D	if	**4**	is correct
E	if	**1, 2, 3, and 4**	are correct

24. Otitis media occurring during the first 6 weeks of life deserves special consideration because the bacteria responsible during this time may be different than in older infants and children. Among these organisms are

(1) *Klebsiella pneumoniae*
(2) *Escherichia coli*
(3) *Pseudomonas aeruginosa*
(4) *Haemophilus influenzae*

25. In addition to characteristic skin lesions, Schönlein-Henoch purpura (anaphylactoid purpura) also is associated with which of the following conditions?

(1) Arthritis
(2) Abdominal pain
(3) Nephritis
(4) Paresis

26. Excessive weight gain in a pregnant woman can indicate the presence of which of the following congenital disorders in the fetus?

(1) Anencephaly
(2) Trisomy 18
(3) Duodenal atresia
(4) Renal agenesis

27. Among those entities that cause enlarged testes after puberty is the "fragile X syndrome." Affected males also present with

(1) precocious puberty
(2) penile enlargement
(3) hormonal changes
(4) mental retardation

28. Plumbism (lead intoxication) can be associated with which of the following hematologic findings?

(1) Decreased activity of delta-aminolevulinic acid dehydratase
(2) Decreased level of erythrocyte protoporphyrin
(3) Increased urinary excretion of protoporphyrin
(4) Increased uptake and utilization of iron

29. At 28 weeks of age a normal baby should be able to

(1) sit with support
(2) roll over
(3) utter repetitive vowel sounds
(4) reach for and grasp large objects

30. Familial dysautonomia (Riley-Day syndrome) is a genetic disease that manifests disturbances in autonomic and sensory functions. This entity is important in the differential diagnosis of a number of chronic problems of childhood, such as

(1) failure to thrive
(2) chronic pulmonary infection
(3) indifference to pain
(4) hypertension

31. Children with cleft palate need to be treated with a team approach if complications are to be avoided. Among the complications that are frequently encountered are

(1) speech disorders
(2) dental caries
(3) malocclusion
(4) otitis media

32. The child pictured below has Down's syndrome. Her surgical scar and purpuric lesions are likely to be consequences of

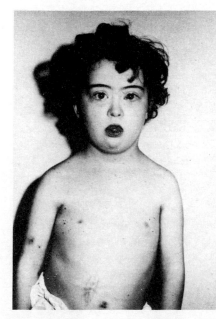

(1) leukemia
(2) thrombotic thrombocytopenic purpura
(3) congenital duodenal atresia
(4) intussusception

33. *Enterobius vermicularis* is a ubiquitous organism that frequently causes more concerns than its medical importance would justify. Among the signs and symptoms that may be related to this parasite's presence are

(1) eosinophilia
(2) anal pruritus
(3) bowel obstruction
(4) sleeplessness

34. Down's syndrome can be seen with which of the following chromosomal patterns?

(1) t(14q21q) centric fusion
(2) 46,XX
(3) Trisomy 21
(4) D/G translocation

35. The infant born to a heroin-addicted mother may show signs of withdrawal as late as 4 to 6 weeks after delivery. The signs of withdrawal may include

(1) flapping tremors
(2) diarrhea
(3) flushing
(4) flaccid extremities

36. The increasing use of organophosphate insecticides has led to a rise in the number of organophosphate poisonings. Physical findings associated with organophosphate intoxication can include

(1) tachycardia
(2) muscle fasciculations
(3) mydriasis
(4) wheezing

SUMMARY OF DIRECTIONS

A	B	C	D	E
1,2,3	1,3	2,4	4	All are
only	only	only	only	correct

37. Among conditions that cause edema of the eyelids is orbital cellulitis, which is a serious infection that must be recognized early and treated aggressively if complications are to be avoided. The condition is usually associated with which of the following?

(1) Chemosis
(2) Normal temperature
(3) Limitation of movement of the eye
(4) Absence of pain

38. Teenage pregnancies and their complications are an increasing problem that calls for a comprehensive approach. In teenage pregnancy there is an increased incidence of

(1) preeclampsia and eclampsia
(2) premature delivery
(3) mental retardation in offspring
(4) nutritional disorders

39. Children who have been abused are likely to develop which of the following?

(1) Fearfulness
(2) Aggressiveness
(3) Hyperactivity
(4) Abusiveness to their own children

40. Whereas in older children the pattern of scabies is similar to that seen in adults, the findings in infants differ in which of the following ways?

(1) Bullae and pustules are common
(2) Burrows are absent
(3) Palms and soles are often involved
(4) Face is spared

41. Anorexia nervosa, which is increasing in frequency, is associated with which of the following symptoms?

(1) Decreased pulse rate
(2) Hyperactivity
(3) Diminished leukocyte count
(4) Increased body temperature

42. Which of the following clinical signs can help differentiate acute otitis externa from acute otitis media?

(1) Pain heightened by movement of the tragus
(2) A red tympanic membrane
(3) Preauricular adenitis
(4) A foul-smelling discharge

43. Type I homocystinemia and Marfan's syndrome have many similar clinical findings, and their ultimate differentiation is sometimes based upon laboratory data. Features associated with both syndromes include

(1) abnormal skeletal appearance
(2) cardiovascular problems
(3) ectopia lentis
(4) mental retardation

DIRECTIONS: Each group of questions below consists of lettered headings followed by a set of numbered items. For each numbered item select the **one** lettered heading with which it is **most** closely associated. Each lettered heading may be used **once, more than once, or not at all.**

Questions 44–48

For each disorder that follows, select the dietary deficiency that is most likely to be responsible.

(A) Caloric deficiency
(B) Thiamine deficiency
(C) Niacin deficiency
(D) Vitamin D deficiency
(E) None of the above

44. Marasmus

45. Kwashiorkor

46. Pellagra

47. Beriberi

48. Rickets

Questions 49–52

For each of the following syndromes that can cause childhood deafness, select the clinical finding with which it is most likely to be associated.

(A) Pulmonary stenosis
(B) White forelock
(C) Goiter
(D) Retinitis pigmentosa
(E) Polydactyly

49. Waardenburg's syndrome

50. Pendred's syndrome

51. Usher's syndrome

52. Leopard syndrome

Questions 53–57

Some of the numerous forms of dwarfism recognizable at birth or within the newborn period have distinguishing features that are useful in differential diagnosis. For each distinguishing feature listed below, select the disorder with which it is most likely to be associated.

(A) Achondrogenesis
(B) Diastrophic dwarfism
(C) Thanatophoric dwarfism
(D) Chondrodystrophia calcificans congenita
(E) Chondroectodermal dysplasia

53. Marked micromelia

54. Congenital heart disease

55. Flattened vertebral bodies

56. Natal teeth

57. Swollen ears

Questions 58–63

Drug and alcohol abuse is a problem that endangers a significant percentage of the adolescent population in the United States. For each of the specific drugs listed below that are currently abused, select the class to which it most likely belongs.

(A) Opiates
(B) Hallucinogens
(C) Intoxicants
(D) Stimulants
(E) Hypnotic sedatives

e 58. Marihuana

R 59. Phencyclidine

C 60. Alcohol

D 61. Cocaine

A 62. Heroin

b 63. Mescaline

Questions 64–67

For each disorder listed below, select the sex and age distribution with which it is most likely to be associated.

(A) Males 4 to 10 years of age
(B) Males 13 to 18 years of age
(C) Females 4 to 10 years of age
(D) Females 10 to 16 years of age
(E) None of the above

A 64. Legg-Calvé-Perthes disease

B 65. Slipped capital femoral epiphysis

D 66. Idiopathic scoliosis

E 67. Subluxation of the head of the radius

Questions 68–72

For poisoning by each substance below, match the treatment most indicated.

(A) Atropine and pralidoxime (2-PAM)
(B) *N*-acetylcysteine (Mucomyst)
(C) Dimercaprol (BAL)
(D) Naloxone (Narcan)
(E) None of the above

C 68. Lead

B 69. Acetaminophen

D 70. Morphine

B 71. Salicylate

A 72. Organophosphate insecticide

Questions 73–75

For poisoning by each substance below, match the treatment most indicated.

(A) Deferoxamine mesylate
(B) Diphenhydramine (Benadryl)
(C) Acetazolamide and sodium bicarbonate
(D) Ethanol
(E) None of the above

B 73. Phenothiazine

A 74. Iron

D 75. Methanol

DIRECTIONS: The group of questions below consists of four lettered headings followed by a set of numbered items. For each numbered item select

A	if the item is associated with	(A) **only**
B	if the item is associated with	(B) **only**
C	if the item is associated with	**both** (A) and (B)
D	if the item is associated with	**neither** (A) nor (B)

Each lettered heading may be used **once, more than once, or not at all.**

Questions 76–82

(A) Aspirin
(B) Acetaminophen
(C) Both
(D) Neither

76. Substantial anti-inflammatory activity

77. Effective analgesic

78. Effective antipyretic

79. Documented to prevent febrile convulsions

80. Hepatotoxic in acute overdosage

81. Frequently used without adequate indication

82. Increased incidence of Reye's syndrome when used in chicken pox and influenza

General Pediatrics

Answers

1. The answer is D. *(Rudolph, ed 17. p 719.)* The percentage of total surface area taken up by the head and neck of a 1-year-old child is almost twice that for the same region in a 10-year-old child and nearly three times that in an adult. The percentage of surface area of the hands, feet, trunk, and genitals remains fairly constant despite the overall increase in total surface area. The surface area of the buttocks is proportionally less in an infant than in an adult.

2. The answer is C. *(Behrman, ed 12. pp 1725–1726.)* Of the three types of lice that are obligate parasites of humans—*Pediculus humanis capitis, Phthirius pubis,* and *Pediculus humanis corporis*—only the body louse, *Pediculus humanis corporis,* is a vector for typhus, trench fever, and relapsing fever. Pediculosis capitis may cause intense pruritus, and secondary infection is common; although the lice may not be seen, the nits may be found attached firmly to hairs, particularly in the occipital region and above the ears. While pediculosis pubis is usually encountered among adolescents, young children may occasionally acquire the disease through close contact. Pediculosis corporis is usually associated with poor hygiene since the lice are most often transmitted via infested clothing or bedding, the nits and lice collecting in the seams. Treatment with gamma benzene hydrochloride, in lotion or shampoo form, is effective for all three types of lice. Clothing and bedding should be carefully laundered.

3. The answer is A. *(Behrman, ed 12. pp 1770–1773.)* The sudden infant death syndrome (SIDS) typically affects infants 2 to 4 months of age and less frequently occurs after 6 months of age. Male infants are affected more frequently than female infants and premature infants more frequently than full-term infants. This syndrome has a higher incidence among infants of drug-addicted mothers and infants who come from socioeconomically deprived families. Siblings of affected infants are more likely to experience crib death than infants in the general population; however, no distinct genetic pattern has been established.

4. The answer is D. *(Behrman, ed 12. pp 1789–1791.)* The initial signs of salicylate poisoning are caused by stimulation of the respiratory center, which increases ventilation and causes the P_{CO_2} to decrease. Salicylate interferes with carbohydrate metabolism and organic acids, mainly lactic acid, are produced as a result of this interference with the Kreb's cycle. The ingested salicylate accounts directly for only a small portion of the acidosis. Salicylate also causes an uncoupling of oxidative phosphorylation, which may cause hyperpyrexia, to which unknowing parents may unfortunately respond with additional salicylates.

5. **The answer is E.** *(Behrman, ed 12. p 172.)* Chronic hypervitaminosis A develops from excessive intake of vitamin A over a period of a month or more. Initial symptoms are nonspecific and include anorexia, pruritus, failure to gain weight, irritability, and tender swelling of bones associated with cortical hyperostosis. Among other manifestations of chronic hypervitaminosis A are hepatomegaly, alopecia, craniotabes, desquamation of palms and soles, seborrheic cutaneous lesions, and signs of increased intracranial pressure, including papilledema and bulging of the fontanelles.

6. **The answer is A.** *(Rudolph, ed 17. p 432.)* Up to 25 percent of girls who have the monoarticular or pauciarticular form of juvenile rheumatoid arthritis have iridocyclitis as their only significant systemic manifestation. Because this eye disorder may require treatment with local or systemic steroids and may develop without signs or symptoms, it is recommended that all children with this form of arthritis have a slit-lamp eye examination every 3 months.

7. **The answer is C.** *(Behrman, ed 12. p 586.)* Lyme disease, named for Lyme, Connecticut, usually presents with erythema chronicum migrans. The rash begins as a small indurated macule or papule on the back, thigh, or buttocks, or occasionally in the axilla. The lesion gradually expands to form a large red ring with central clearing; subsequently, other similar lesions may occur. The lesions are usually warm and although generally painless occasionally produce a painful burning sensation. The rash usually lasts about 3 weeks but may last from just a few days to 8 weeks.

Attacks of arthritis, particularly involving the knees and other large joints, may last for months and often recur. Fever, aseptic meningitis, myocardial conduction defects, and cranial nerve palsies may also occur. Treatment is with penicillin, or tetracycline in the patient over 12 years of age.

8. **The answer is C.** *(Rudolph, ed 17. pp 1542–1543.)* In human somatic cells, only one X chromosome in each cell is genetically active. The additional X chromosomes become inactivated and condensed; these are visible within the nuclei of interphase cells as sex-chromatin bodies (Barr bodies). Thus, the number of sex-chromatin bodies in a cell is one less than the total number of X chromosomes.

Microscopic examination of a buccal smear from a normal female (XX) therefore shows one Barr body in the cell nucleus, as shown below:

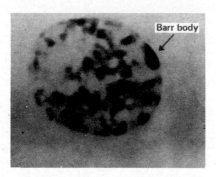

9. The answer is E. *(Rudolph, ed 17. p 1216.)* Paraphimosis occurs when a retracted prepuce with phimosis remains behind the glans; edema develops, hindering reduction of the paraphimosis. This disorder can lead to gangrene of the glans. Reduction of the paraphimosis by pressure on the glans and traction on the prepuce usually necessitates sedation; slitting of the constricting ring or circumcision may be required. Phimosis is characterized by an inability to retract the foreskin of the penis after the age of 3 years because of a narrowing of the preputial opening. Balanitis and balanoposthitis are inflammatory disorders affecting the glans penis and, in the case of balanoposthitis, the prepuce; these disorders develop when persistent adhesions between the foreskin and glans penis cause retention of smegma mixed with urine and lead to infection or chemical irritation.

10. The answer is B. *(Rudolph, ed 17. pp 327–328.)* Familial hypercholesterolemia (classic type II hyperlipoproteinemia) is the most common form of familial hyperlipidemia occurring in childhood. It is transmitted as an autosomal dominant trait. The incidence of affected heterozygotes has been estimated at between 0.2 and 0.5 percent of the population. The disorder is characterized by elevation of total cholesterol as well as low-density lipoprotein cholesterol levels in the plasma. Manifestations of familial hypercholesterolemia include the presence of tendon xanthomas, an increased likelihood of premature ischemic heart disease, and development during childhood of corneal arcus. Although a heterozygous child may be asymptomatic up to the age of ten, homozygous children may have physical signs, particularly planar xanthomas, from birth.

11. The answer is D. *(Behrman, ed 12. p 1622.)* Osgood-Schlatter disease is most probably due to repeated trauma to the tibial tuberosity caused by excessive use of the quadriceps muscle. The disease causes pain and swelling over the tibial tubercle and tenderness on palpation. Irregular mineralization of the tibial tubercle is usually visible on x-ray. Avoidance of strenuous activity for 1 to 2 months is usually sufficient treatment. If this does not control symptoms, a cast may be required.

12. The answer is E. *(Silverman, p 156.)* According to the International Code of Ethics for Biomedical Research, the subject of human experimentation must be informed that he or she can withdraw from the study at **any** time. In addition, concern for the interests of the subject must always prevail over the interests of science and society. The investigation should cease if hazards arise that outweigh the potential benefits.

13. The answer is D. *(Silverman, pp 127–138.)* The probability given is the estimation of the odds that the observed differences could have occurred by chance alone. The interpretation of these results depends on an assessment of such factors in study design as the size of the sample and the type of controls used, and on the severity of the disease, the side effects, and the importance of the treatment. The tendency for negative results to remain unpublished should also be kept in mind.

14. The answer is A. *(Gilman, ed 7. p 10.)* Chemically equivalent drugs meet the same chemical and physical standards. They are biologically equivalent if they result in similar concentrations in the body and may be called therapeutically equivalent if this equivalence has been demonstrated by a clinical trial. It could also be said that they are equal in bioavailability. Equivalence is a particular problem with the oral form of a slowly absorbed drug such as digoxin.

15. The answer is C. *(Behrman, ed 12. pp 539–547. Finberg, pp 206-211.)* Children in acute and obvious distress because of an episode of asthma usually respond to treatment with subcutaneous epinephrine. Two or three injections may be required before symptoms are relieved. Once their asthmatic episodes have abated, affected children may be given a long-acting form of epinephrine, such as crystalline epinephrine suspension, before going home. Theophylline toxicity should be suspected in children who develop vomiting, irritability, or seizures, and xanthine administration should cease until serum theophylline measurements can be obtained. Sedatives, which may cause respiratory depression, are contraindicated in the treatment of children with respiratory distress. Antibiotics are generally not indicated unless specific signs of infection such as high fever, elevated white cell count with increased neutrophils, or signs of pneumonia are present. Excess fluid should not be administered for fear of producing pulmonary edema. N-acetyl cysteine and cromolyn should not be given since they are likely to make bronchospasm worse.

16. The answer is E. *(Behrman, ed 12. pp 1693–1694.)* Pityriasis rosea is of unknown etiology. The lesions may be asymptomatic to severely pruritic. The characteristic "herald patch" usually precedes the general eruption by 5 to 10 days and is a large, solitary, round or oval scaly lesion occurring anywhere on the body.

When the generalized eruption occurs, it involves mainly the trunk and proximal limbs. These lesions are usually scaly, less than 1 cm in diameter, oval or round, and pink to brown. The long axis of each lesion is aligned with the cutaneous cleavage lines, which may form a "christmas tree" pattern on the patient's trunk. The eruption usually lasts 2 to 12 weeks. There is no specific therapy and treatment is symptomatic.

17. The answer is C. *(Behrman, ed 12. p 1555.)* Beyond the newborn period there should be no red blood cells in the CSF. Their presence may be due to a traumatic lumbar puncture or to a recent subarachnoid hemorrhage. With subarachnoid hemorrhage, the supernatant is xanthochromic and the collecting tubes successively show equal quantities of RBCs. With traumatic taps there is usually gradual clearing of the RBCs as successive tubes are used and the supernatant is colorless on centrifugation. In the newborn infant up to 15 leukocytes and 500 RBCs may normally be present and the protein level may be as high as 100 mg/dl. By three months of age the protein level should have fallen below 30 mg/dl.

18. The answer is B. *(Rudolph, ed 17. pp 745–746.)* The three chelating agents used in the United States to treat individuals who have plumbism are edetate calcium disodium (Ca EDTA), dimercaprol (British anti-lewisite), and D-penicillamine. In children having the highest soft-tissue lead content (i.e., those who have acute encephalopathy), chelating agents must be administered in molar amounts in excess of those of the ingested lead—otherwise, the lead may once again disseminate within tissues of the body and cause further toxicity. Both edetate calcium disodium and dimercaprol should be given promptly in the treatment of a child affected with acute lead encephalopathy; D-penicillamine may be administered later during therapy. Careful administration of parenteral fluids is necessary so that further increase in cerebral edema does not occur.

19. The answer is E. *(Behrman, ed 12. pp 1089–1090.)* The sweat test remains the most reliable test for cystic fibrosis. In children, chloride levels in sweat that are greater than 60 mEq/L are diagnostic of cystic fibrosis; sodium concentrations are approximately 10 mEq/L higher. Results of sweat tests in adults may be harder to interpret, because sweat electrolyte concentrations normally are higher in adults than in children. The mechanism governing this alteration of sweat electrolyte levels is unknown. Glycogen storage disease, vasopressin-resistant diabetes insipidus, untreated adrenal insufficiency, and a type of ectodermal dysplasia are among the rare conditions that also may be associated with elevation of sweat electrolyte concentrations; none of these conditions, however, is likely to be confused clinically with cystic fibrosis.

20. The answer is B. *(Behrman, ed 12. pp 1086–1099.)* It is believed that cystic fibrosis is inherited as an autosomal recessive trait, and statistical evidence exists to support this contention. As a result, each child born to parents who have had one child with cystic fibrosis has a 25-percent chance of being affected, a 50-percent chance of being a carrier, and a 25-percent chance of not carrying the gene (or genes) at all. Heterozygotes (carriers) for cystic fibrosis are clinically asymptomatic.

21. The answer is B. *(Rudolph, ed 17. pp 359–360.)* Achondroplasia, occurring with an incidence of approximately 1 in every 9000 deliveries, is the most common form of skeletal dysplasia. Affected individuals bear a striking resemblance to one another and are identified by their extremely short extremities, prominent foreheads, short, stubby fingers, and a marked lumbar lordosis. Although they go through normal puberty, affected females must have children by cesarean section because of an associated pelvic deformity.

22. The answer is E. *(Behrman, ed 12. pp 360–361.)* The clavicle is the bone most frequently fractured during delivery. This usually occurs when the shoulder is difficult to deliver during vertex presentation or during the delivery of an extended arm in breech presentation. Typically, the infant does not move the arm on the side of the fracture and there may be crepitation and irregularity over the fracture site. There may be spasm of the sternocleidomastoid on the side of the fracture, and swelling may obliterate the usually present supraclavicular depression. These fractures often develop a great deal of callus formation within a week. The outcome is very good and treatment is usually simple immobilization of shoulder and arm on the involved side.

23. The answer is B. *(AAP-CAPP, ed 2. pp 3-5.)* Milk is advised for caustic and irritant ingestions when endoscopy is not to be done quickly. It is not recommended to be given along with ipecac since it delays the onset of vomiting. Milk decreases the efficiency of activated charcoal and should not be given with it. Activated charcoal should be diluted with water and kept stirred during drinking and is best taken through a straw.

24. The answer is E (all). *(Behrman, ed 12. p 409.)* The symptoms of otitis media in the newborn are similar to those of sepsis: poor feeding, lethargy, vomiting, jaundice, irritability, or low fever. The diagnosis is difficult because of the narrow external ear canal and may be based only on decreased mobility of the eardrum. In addition to the pathogens ordinarily associated with acute otitis media in older infants and children (*H. influenzae* and *S. pneumoniae*), *S. aureus,* group B streptococci, *E. coli, K. pneumoniae,* and *P. aeruginosa* are commonly found in infected newborns under 6 weeks old. Therapy with an appropriate oral antibiotic may be given if the infant can be observed closely. However, if sepsis is also suspected, parenteral therapy with ampicillin and an aminoglycoside is necessary until culture results become available.

25. The answer is E (all). *(Behrman, ed 12. pp 1338–1340.)* The clinical manifestations of Schönlein-Henoch purpura are due to vasculitis. Acute inflammation in the skin causes characteristic lesions that begin as urticarial wheals or red maculopapules and progress to purpura, usually on the buttocks and legs. An exudate containing lymphocytes, polymorphonuclear leukocytes, eosinophils, and red blood cells tends to accumulate around the small blood vessels of the corium. Inflammation and hemorrhage also may occur at other sites, notably joints, kidneys, the gastrointestinal tract, and the central nervous system. The arthritis associated with Schönlein-Henoch purpura usually involves the larger joints, particularly the knees and ankles. Nephritis can develop and lead to chronic renal disease, and gastrointestinal involvement, although usually limited to colicky abdominal pain and bleeding, rarely includes intussusception.

26. The answer is A (1, 2, 3). *(Behrman, ed 12. pp 317, 330.)* It is generally presumed that duodenal atresia leads to hydramnios (polyhydramnios) by interference with reabsorption of swallowed amniotic fluid. Abnormal production or release of antidiuretic hormone by fetuses who have anomalies of the central nervous system is considered to be responsible for hydramnios during their gestations. Hydramnios also is associated with approximately 80 percent of infants who have trisomy 18. Oligohydramnios occurs in association with congenital abnormalities of the fetal kidneys, such as renal agenesis, that inhibit formation of fetal urine.

27. The answer is D (4). *(Behrman, ed 12. pp 1500–1501.)* An association between mental retardation and enlargement of testes occurs in the "fragile X syndrome." The testes reach 30 to 40 ml in size after puberty, the penis is of normal size, and there are no known hormonal changes. Many of these patients have a fragile site at the end of the long arm of the X chromosome. In these families it is important to identify affected boys by chromosomal analysis in order to do genetic counseling.

28. The answer is B (1, 3). *(Rudolph, ed 17. p 741.)* Lead disrupts the production of hemoglobin by inhibiting several steps in the manufacture of heme. In addition to decreased activity of delta-aminolevulinic acid dehydratase and increased excretion of delta-aminolevulinic acid in the urine, lead poisoning leads to increased erythrocyte protoporphyrin levels and decreased uptake and utilization of iron. Lead also interferes with the synthesis of globin in maturing erythrocytes. As a result of these impairments, a hypochromic, microcytic anemia ensues and basophilic stippling of red blood cells occurs. Red blood cell survival time is shortened and a very mild hemolytic anemia may result.

29. The answer is E (all). *(Behrman, ed 12. pp 16–19.)* A 28-week-old infant should be able to sit briefly with pelvic support, roll over, reach for and hold large objects, and utter vowel sounds. At 40 weeks of age, an infant should creep or crawl, sit up without support, and make consonant sounds in a repetitive fashion ("dada," "mama"). At about 1 year, infants generally are able to walk with assistance. Evaluation of a child's development can be affected by a variety of circumstances, such as hunger, fatigue, or illness, that can impede a child's performance. Serial examinations are therefore much more reliable in assessing accurately a child's development.

30. The answer is E (all). *(Behrman, ed 12. pp 1598–1599.)* The Riley-Day syndrome, inherited as autosomal recessive, is most common in Ashkenazi Jews and has a variety of clinical manifestations. Poor coordination of swallowing movements may lead to repeated episodes of vomiting, gagging, and aspiration. The aspirations may set the stage for repeated pulmonary infections with eventual development of chronic pulmonary failure, which is the most common cause of death. Other manifestations of autonomic system dysfunction include increased sweating, labile hypertension, orthostatic hypotension, and poor temperature control. Disturbances in pain sensation lead to repeated trauma, and absence of corneal sensation increases the chances for development of corneal ulceration. The diagnosis is suggested by the finding of a smooth tongue, which is a result of diminished or absent taste buds. There is also no production of the characteristic flare when the histamine skin test is performed. There is no specific treatment, but the control of respiratory infections and the prevention of aspiration, corneal ulceration (with artificial tears), dehydration, and injuries are advisable.

31. The answer is E (all). *(Behrman, ed 12. pp 881–882.)* The incidence of isolated cleft palate is approximately 1 in every 2,500 births. The incidence of cleft lip, with or without cleft palate, is approximately 1 in every 1,000 births. Speech defects can result or persist even after adequate surgical closure of the palate cleft. They are due to a failure of the palatal and pharyngeal muscular structures to produce an adequate valve between the nasopharynx and the oropharynx. Therefore, not enough pressure is built up to produce certain sounds, such as "s," "sh," and "ch." This valve mechanism also fails to be brought into play during swallowing, thus preventing adequate closure of the eustachian tube, which makes the development of otitis media and subsequent hearing problems a persistent problem for many of these children. Dental caries are also a major problem for these children and require constant surveillance. A team approach is needed to treat adequately the comprehensive needs of these children.

32. The answer is B (1,3). *(Behrman, ed 12. pp 295–299.)* Down's syndrome is a major cause of mental retardation. Affected children show moderate to severe retardation and have a variety of morphologic abnormalities. A small, flattened skull, outwardly and upwardly sloping palpebral fissures, the presence of epicanthic folds, and a protruding tongue contribute to their characteristic facies. These children have a higher incidence of duodenal atresia, which requires surgical correction to relieve intestinal obstruction. Children who have Down's syndrome also have a higher incidence of congenital heart disease. First signs of leukemia, which is 10 to 20 times more likely to occur in Down's syndrome children than in the general population, may be petechiae and bruises, which occur because the uncontrolled proliferation of leukocytes in the bone marrow suppresses platelet production.

33. The answer is C (2,4). *(Behrman, ed 12. p 858.)* Enterobius vermicularis (pinworm) infestation occurs in all regions of the world and particularly affects children between the ages of 5 and 14 years. Humans are infested by the ingestion of eggs carried under fingernails or in bedding, house dust, or food. The eggs hatch in the stomach and the larvae migrate to the cecal region where they become adult worms. The females migrate at night to the perianal region and deposit their eggs, leading to sleeplessness and itching. Diagnosis is made by discovery of eggs or worms upon microscopic examination of transparent adhesive tape pressed against the perianal area before waking. Although cleanliness is important, there is no proof that it plays a role in the control of the pinworms. Much of the social anxiety needs to be down-played as the infestation is essentially harmless. There is no tissue invasion nor is eosinophilia noted. A single dose of mebendazole is recommended therapy.

34. The answer is E (all). *(Rudolph, ed 17. pp 242–243. Behrman, ed 12. pp 295–299.)* Children who have Down's syndrome most commonly have trisomy 21; translocations, especially between D-group and G-group chromosomes—t(14q21q) centric fusion is the most common of these abnormalities—account for a small percentage of cases. Children who have trisomy 21, which is caused by nondisjunction, have 47 chromosomes; karyotypes of children with a translocation reveal a normal chromosome count of 46. The chromosomal defect causing translocation Down's syndrome can be carried by asymptomatic individuals if the translocation is balanced (i.e., if the amount of chromosomal material is normal, regardless of structural changes in the chromosomes). Therefore, chromosome analysis should be performed because the chance that future siblings will have Down's syndrome is significantly greater if translocation rather than nondisjunction is the etiology.

35. The answer is A (1,2,3). *(Behrman, ed 12. pp 394–395.)* The great majority of infants born to mothers addicted to heroin show clinical manifestations of withdrawal within the first 48 hours after birth; some, however, present as late as 4 to 6 weeks of age. The infants are very irritable and usually have tremors that may be fine but are often coarse and flapping. Their extremities are hyperreflexic and stiff. They may have a high-pitched cry, diarrhea, myoclonic jerks, and convulsions. The diagnosis is usually a clinical one based on history and symptoms. Treatment using a variety of regimens has been successful.

36. The answer is C (2,4). *(Rudolph, ed 17. pp 735–737.)* When the clinical signs of constricted pupils, bradycardia, and muscle fasciculations are associated with the sudden onset of neurological symptoms, progressive respiratory distress, diaphoresis, diarrhea, and overabundant salivation, a diagnosis of organophosphate poisoning should be suspected. Intake of organophosphate agents can occur by ingestion, inhalation, or absorption through skin or mucosa. Organophosphates inhibit carboxylic esterase enzymes, including acetylcholinesterase and pseudocholinesterase; toxicity depends primarily on the inactivation or inhibition of acetylcholinesterase.

Treatment consists of gastric lavage, if the poison has been ingested, or decontamination of the skin, if exposure has been through contact; maintenance of adequate ventilation and fluid and electrolyte balance also is indicated. All symptomatic children should receive atropine and, if severely affected, cholinesterase reactivating oximes as well. Cholinesterase reactivating oximes quickly restore consciousness by inhibiting the muscarine- and nicotine-like synaptic actions of acetylcholine. One cholinesterase reactivating oxime is pralidoxime chloride (Protopam).

37. The answer is B (1,3). *(Behrman, ed 12. pp 1767–1768.)* Orbital cellulitis is a serious infection of the tissues of the orbit and is characterized by edema of the conjunctivae, proptosis, limitation of movement of the eye, erythema and swelling of the eyelids, pain, and systemic signs such as fever. Orbital cellulitis may follow directly from a wound or bacteremia, but the most common path is by extension from the paranasal sinuses. The organisms most frequently involved as pathogens are *Haemophilus influenzae, Staphylococcus aureus,* group A beta-hemolytic streptococci, and *Streptococcus pneumoniae.* The risk of complications—including loss of vision, cavernous sinus thrombosis, meningitis, or brain abscess—is great. Prompt hospitalization and parenteral antibiotic therapy is indicated.

38. The answer is E (all). *(Behrman, ed 12. pp 61–62.)* The main obstetric complications of teenage pregnancy are preeclampsia and eclampsia, which are thought to be due to inadequate prenatal care and nutrition. The rate of prematurity is high, and this in turn is thought to account for the increased incidence of mental retardation among children of teenage mothers. The incidence of repeat pregnancy is high, and too few communities make provisions for the mother to continue her education. A combination of medical, social, psychological, and educational resources must be made available to permit optimum health and development of the teenage mother and her child.

39. The answer is E (all). *(Behrman, ed 12. pp 99–105.)* Battered children may be more permanently wounded psychologically than physically. Children who have been abused may be fearful of personal closeness, aggressive, and hyperactive.

Tendencies toward provocative and impulsive behavior also are common, and abused children may subsequently abuse their own children. It is imperative that physicians recognize that these factors may contribute to additional physical and psychological injuries and that the provoking child may urgently need psychological assessment and therapy.

40. The answer is A (1,2,3). *(Behrman, ed 12. pp 1723–1725).* Scabies, caused by the mite *Sarcoptes scabiei* var. *hominis,* has recently been increasing among all age groups. Most older children and adults present with intensely pruritic wheals, papules, vesicles and threadlike burrows in the interdigital areas, groin, elbows, and ankles; the palms, soles, face, and head are spared. However, infants usually present with bullae and pustules and the areas spared in adults are often involved in infants. Because of the potential neurotoxic effect to infants of gamma benzene hexachloride through percutaneous absorption, an alternative should be used, such as 10% crotamiton lotion or cream or a 6% sulfur ointment.

41. The answer is A (1,2,3). *(Rudolph, ed 17. p 72.)* Anorexia nervosa, a life-threatening disorder that primarily affects preadolescent and adolescent girls, is characterized by profound weight loss (25 to 30 percent or more of body weight). Despite vigorous investigation, no organic basis has been found. Affected individuals have a distorted body image and are preoccupied with food. Body temperature may be as low as 35.6°C (96°F); pulse rate, blood pressure, and leukocyte count also are decreased. Anorectic individuals are hyperactive and expend a tremendous amount of energy. Therapy is difficult; skillful psychotherapeutic management is fundamental.

42. The answer is B (1,3). *(Behrman, ed 12. pp 1024–1025.)* The pain of otitis externa but not of otitis media is increased by movement of the tragus. In addition, the presence of preauricular, postauricular, or cervical adenitis, a feature of outer-ear but not middle-ear disease, aids in making the proper diagnosis. The tympanic membrane, if visualized in otitis externa, may appear normal or red; a red tympanic membrane also characterizes acute suppurative otitis media. The presence of a foul-smelling discharge may occur in association with either otitis externa or otitis media, following rupture of a tympanic membrane.

43. The answer is A (1,2,3). *(Behrman, ed 12. pp 428–429, 1167.)* About 50 percent of individuals with type I homocystinemia are mentally retarded, but this is not found in patients with Marfan's syndrome. They both tend to develop dislocation of the lens and a peculiar tall body habitus, with especially long, thin, tapering extremities. Cardiovascular problems are common to both. With homocystinemia, individuals may develop thromboembolic episodes because of abnormalities in intravascular clotting. Those with Marfan's syndrome often have progressive aortic dilatation with medial cystic necrosis, resulting in aortic insufficiency and dissecting aneurysm, which is often the cause of death. Patients with homocystinemia can be detected by the presence of homocystine in the urine by the cyanide-nitroprusside test. Type I homocystinemia is due to deficiency of the enzyme cystathionine synthase. Some of these patients with type I homocystinemia respond to large doses of vitamin B_6 and to methionine restriction.

44–48. The answers are: 44-A, 45-E, 46-C, 47-B, 48-D. *(Behrman, ed 12. pp 166–168, 172–175, 1653–1656.)* Marasmus (infantile atrophy) is due to inadequate caloric intake that may be linked with such factors as insufficient food resources, poor feeding techniques, metabolic disorders, and congenital anomalies. Patients with marasmus have progressive weight loss, constipation, muscular atrophy, loss of skin turgor, hypothermia, and possibly edema. In advanced disease, affected infants are lethargic and may have starvation diarrhea, with small, mucus-containing stools.

Kwashiorkor, which is caused by a severe deficiency of protein, is the most common—and most serious—type of malnutrition in the world. Caloric intake in affected children may be adequate. Children who have protein deficiency become more susceptible to infection; vomiting, diarrhea, muscle wasting, dermatitis, hepatosplenomegaly, edema, dyspigmentation of the skin and hair, and changes in mental status are among the many manifestations of this disease. The most important laboratory finding is a decrease in serum albumin level.

Pellagra, which literally means "rough skin," is due to a deficiency of niacin (nicotinic acid). Niacin is an essential component of two enzymes—nicotinamide adenine dinucleotide (NAD) and nicotinamide adenine dinucleotide phosphate (NADP)—that are needed for electron transfer and glycolysis. Pellagra is most prevalent in areas that rely on corn as a basic foodstuff (corn contains little tryptophan, which can be converted into niacin). The classic ("3-D") triad of clinical symptoms of pellagra consists of dermatitis, diarrhea, and dementia.

Beriberi results from a deficiency of thiamine (vitamin B_1), which is essential for the synthesis of acetylcholine and for the operation of certain enzyme systems in carbohydrate metabolism. Thiamine is present in fair amounts in cereals, fruits, vegetables, and eggs; meat and legumes are good sources. Thiamine is destroyed by heat, and polishing of grains reduces their thiamine content by removing the coverings that contain most of the vitamin. Clinical disturbances stemming from thiamine deficiency are congestive heart failure, peripheral neuritis, and psychic disturbances.

Rickets is a disorder of growing bone characterized by defective mineralization of matrix. Rickets that responds to administration of physiological doses of vitamin D is termed vitamin D-deficient rickets. Deficiency of vitamin D can lead to osseous changes, such as enlargement of the costochondral junctions ("rachitic rosary") and craniotabes, within a few months; advanced rickets may cause scoliosis, pelvic and leg deformities, "pigeon breast," rachitic dwarfism, and other disorders.

49–52. The answers are: 49-B, 50-C, 51-D, 52-A. *(Rudolph, ed 17. p. 891.)* Waardenburg's syndrome is the most common of several syndromes that are characterized by both deafness and pigmentary changes. Features of this syndrome, which is inherited as an autosomal dominant disorder, include a distinctive white forelock, heterochromia irides, unilateral or bilateral congenital deafness, and lateral displacement of the inner canthi.

Individuals who have Pendred's syndrome, inherited as an autosomal recessive trait, typically have a marked hearing loss and thyroid dysfunction. Goiter, which usually develops before affected children reach the age of 10 years, may arise because their thyroid glands are unable to convert inorganic iodine into organic iodine. The benign goiter responds to thyroid replacement therapy.

Congenital deafness is also a symptom of the autosomal recessive Usher's syndrome. Pigmentary changes in the retina (retinitis pigmentosa) can be detected in affected infants, and these degenerative changes continue throughout life. Early visual impairments include loss of night vision and development of tunnel vision. Functional blindness can arise in affected adolescents and adults.

Leopard syndrome is characterized by the presence of multiple **l**entigines, **o**cular hypertelorism, **p**ulmonary stenosis, **a**bnormal genitalia, **r**etardation of growth, and profound **d**eafness. The syndrome is inherited as an autosomal dominant disorder with variable penetrance.

53–57. The answers are: 53-A, 54-E, 55-C, 56-E, 57-B. *(Behrman, ed 12. pp 1637–1641.)* Achondrogenesis is a lethal chondrodystrophy that is associated with severe micromelia, a relatively large head, and a narrow trunk.

Diastrophic dwarfism, another type of short-limbed dwarfism, is distinguishable by the swelling of the pinna that appears within the first 3 weeks of life and persists for 3 to 4 weeks, leaving the ears with thick, firm, deformed cartilage. The disease is inherited as an autosomal recessive trait and intelligence is normal in affected children.

Chondrodystrophia calcificans congenita (Conradi's disease) is frequently associated with cataracts and optic atrophy. Children with this disease may also suffer from seborrheic dermatitis or ichthyosiform erythroderma. The radiologic finding of discrete, multiple calcified densities in those bones formed in hyaline cartilage helps to establish the diagnosis.

Children with thanatophoric dwarfism are born with hypotonia and rapidly develop respiratory distress and asphyxia from severe narrowing of the thorax. Characteristic x-ray findings include marked flattening of the vertebral bodies.

Chondroectodermal dysplasia (Ellis–van Creveld syndrome) has an unusually high incidence among the Amish, although cases among non-Amish people have also been reported. Anomalies occur in these children in all the embryonic layers of development. Ectodermal abnormalities include fine, sparse hair, dystrophic nails, and peg-shaped teeth with abnormal spacing. Natal teeth are frequently present. Mesodermal abnormalities are manifested by bone involvement resulting in dwarfism, congenital heart disease, and renal malformation. Polydactylism is usually present in these children, who have normal intelligence. The disease has an autosomal recessive inheritance. Penetrance is variable and may be manifested by polydactyly as an isolated finding.

58–63. The answers are: 58-C, 59-B, 60-C, 61-D, 62-A, 63-B. *(Behrman, ed 12. pp 1524–1529.)* In 1972, the National Commission on Marihuana and Drug Abuse reported that 7 percent of American youths were regular users of marihuana. Users of this drug may exhibit a variety of behavioral changes from simple euphoria to hallucinations. Users' response time and coordination may be impaired. A 1976 survey revealed that there seemed to be no increase in usage of marihuana in adolescents but that alcohol was assuming greater importance as an additive substance.

Phencyclidine (PCP, angel dust) is one of the more common hallucinogens available on the "street." Because PCP may cause confusion and a wide variety of hallucinations, it is of especially high risk to individuals prone to psychiatric problems, in whom prolonged psychosis may be produced. Lysergic acid diethylamide (LSD) and PCP are often the active ingredients in substances sold as mescaline or psilocybin because they are relatively easy to produce.

Alcohol, while regarded by many as simply a beverage, is an intoxicant that, among other problems, accounts for an increasing number of automobile accidents. It has been reported that as many as 28 percent of adolescents in the United States are problem drinkers.

Cocaine is a stimulant that is increasingly available. Formerly, cocaine was used in combination with heroin, but it is now often used as a primary drug, even though it is very expensive. Dealing in drugs may be the easiest way for an adolescent to meet the cost of drug use.

Heroin, along with methadone and morphine, is an opiate. It is usually injected but occasionally is taken intranasally. Infections at the injection site, hepatitis, endocarditis, and tetanus are among the medical problems encountered in opiate users.

Mescaline, another hallucinogen, is more likely to be LSD or PCP. Prolonged use of hallucinogens may result in disturbed interpersonal relations, poor time and place orientation, and regressive behavior. With abstinence, hallucinogenic flashbacks may recur for months.

64–67. The answers are: 64-A, 65-B, 66-D, 67-E. *(Behrman, ed 12. pp 1620–1621, 1624–1625, 1629. Rudolph, ed 17. pp 1834–1837.)* Legg-Calvé-Perthes disease (coxa plana) is aseptic necrosis and flattening of the femoral head; the cause of this disorder is unknown. Boys between the ages of 4 and 10 years are most frequently affected. Presenting symptoms include a limp, pain in the knee or hip, or limitation of weight bearing.

Slipped capital femoral epiphysis occurs typically in adolescents; the disorder is most common among obese boys. The etiology is unknown. Onset of this disorder is gradual; pain referred to the knee is characteristic and may mask the hip pathology.

Idiopathic scoliosis occurs most frequently in adolescent girls and requires prompt evaluation. Treatment by bracing, spinal fusion, or both is sometimes necessary. Unrecognized prior infection of the nervous system, leading to muscle weakness, may be a factor in some cases of idiopathic scoliosis.

Subluxation of the head of the radius occurs most commonly in children who are two to five years of age and have been jerked forcibly by the hand. Affected children have pain in the elbow and are unable to supinate the forearm. The diagnosis is established if supination of the forearm, while the elbow is stabilized, corrects the subluxation.

68–72. The answers are: 68-C, 69-B, 70-D, 71-E, 72-A. *(AAP-CAPP, ed 2. pp 22–25, 86–92, 108–110, 112–114, 126–130, 141–150. Finberg, pp 201–204.)* The most important aspect of the management of lead poisoning is identification and withdrawal of the source of the lead. Patients with symptomatic lead poisoning or high lead levels in the blood (over 100 mcg per 100 ml) should be treated with both dimercaprol and calcium EDTA. With milder poisoning calcium EDTA alone may be used.

Acetaminophen poisoning produces hepatotoxicity with the possibility of hepatic failure and death at overdoses beginning at 140 mg/kg. There may be a latent period of several days between ingestion and onset of symptoms and signs of illness. Emesis should be induced or gastic lavage should be started as early as possible, but activated charcoal should be avoided since this will interfere with the action of N-acetylcysteine, which should be given as early as possible and acts by removing the hepatotoxic metabolite.

Morphine and other narcotics produce their major toxic effect by suppression of ventilation. Ventilatory support may be necessary initially, but naloxone is a specific antidote and may be very rapidly effective. The effect of naloxone may wear off more quickly than the effects of the drug for which it was given, so careful observation and repeated doses may be necessary.

Salicylate poisoning is not treated with any of these drugs. It produces metabolic acidosis and respiratory alkalosis, hyperglycemia and hypoglycemia, confusion, convulsions, coma, cardiorespiratory failure, and possibly death. Excretion of salicylates in the urine can be markedly enhanced by the administration of acetazolamide and intravenous sodium bicarbonate.

Organophosphate insecticides are absorbed from all sites and act by inhibiting cholinesterases, which leads to excessively high levels of acetylcholine, thus affecting the parasympathetic nervous system, muscle, and the central nervous system. Health workers, protecting themselves with rubber gloves and taking care to avoid contact with contaminated skin or clothing, should wash the pesticide from the skin, induce emesis or perform gastic lavage, support ventilation, and administer atropine followed by pralidoxime (2-PAM).

73–75. The answers are: 73-B, 74-A, 75-D. *(AAP-CAPP, ed 2. pp 75–80, 101–103, 117–120, 141–150.)* Phenothiazine toxicity is particularly common in infants and children, and with dehydration and fever. Extrapyramidal symptoms such as oculogyric crisis, tremors, and dysphagia may occur even with small doses. These dystonic symptoms respond surprisingly quickly to the intravenous or intramuscular administration of diphenhydramine (Benadryl). More severe poisoning with vasomotor collapse, convulsions, coma or respiratory failure requires intensive care.

Iron in the form of salts such as ferrous sulfate or ferrous gluconate used to treat iron deficiency anemia may be highly toxic to infants; as few as three tablets may cause severe symptoms and as few as nine tablets may be lethal to young children. Symptoms occur in two phases: gastrointestinal symptoms such as bloody vomiting or diarrhea and abdominal pain, followed by a latent period of up to 2 days, and terminating with cardiovascular collapse. Deferoxamine given intravenously or intramuscularly complexes with the iron and is excreted in the urine, to which it imparts the color of vin rose.

Methanol, also known as methyl alcohol or wood alcohol, is present in window-washer fluid, paint remover, and as the alcohol in gasohol. Toxicity is produced by its hepatic metabolites, formaldehyde and formic acid, which cause a profound metabolic acidosis. Treatment includes emptying the stomach by inducing emesis or by gastic lavage, the intravenous infusion of ethanol to saturate the enzyme systems that convert methanol to toxins, and in severe poisoning the use of hemodialysis to remove the methanol.

76–82. The answers are: 76-A, 77-C, 78-C, 79-D, 80-B, 81-C, 82-A. *(Gilman, ed 7. pp 680–689, 692–695.)* Aspirin and acetaminophen are used in vast quantities in treating infants and children, often with essentially no appropriate indication, even by physicians. High fever (over 106°F) can damage the brain and other organs, but the usual temperatures of fever for which these drugs are frequently used have not been shown to be harmful and may even be helpful. The reason for the prevalent fever phobia is not clear.

These drugs have not been shown to prevent febrile convulsions. Both drugs are effective antipyretics. While aspirin has an anti-inflammatory effect, acetaminophen does not. This anti-inflammatory effect relieves symptoms, but the influence on the course of such diseases as rheumatic fever or osteoarthritis is unclear, although there is some recent evidence that it may improve the outlook for Kawasaki syndrome.

Both drugs are effective analgesics and both are toxic in overdosage, but only acetaminophen is primarily hepatotoxic. The acute toxic oral dose of acetaminophen is 140 mg/kg, which is slightly below the toxic dosage of aspirin. Aspirin poisoning was much more common before the introduction of legislation requiring child-proof containers. Aspirin has been implicated in the etiology of Reye's syndrome when given to patients with influenza or chicken pox. Regulations now require a statement, printed on the product, warning of this problem.

The Newborn Infant

DIRECTIONS: Each question below contains five suggested responses. Select the **one best** response to each question.

83. A contraindication to breast feeding is

(A) cesarean delivery
(B) low birth weight
(C) hospitalization of the infant
(D) administration of radioactive isotopes to the mother
(E) small breasts

84. Whole cow's milk as an infant feeding always supplies more than adequate amounts of

(A) protein
(B) iron
(C) linoleic acid
(D) vitamin C
(E) water

85. A full-term newborn infant is having episodes of cyanosis and apnea, which are worse when he is attempting to feed, but he seems better when he is crying. The most important diagnosis to establish quickly is

(A) ventricular septal defect
(B) Ondine's curse (primary alveolar hypoventilation syndrome)
(C) choanal atresia
(D) sickle cell anemia
(E) floppy palate syndrome

86. A 2-week-old infant has had no immunizations, sleeps 18 hours a day, weighs 3.5 kg, takes 60 ml of standard infant formula four times a day, but no solid food, and takes no iron or vitamin supplements. Of most concern is

(A) immunization status
(B) caloric intake
(C) circadian rhythm
(D) iron levels
(E) levels of vitamins A, C, and D

87. In a neonate who has asphyxia, all the following sequelae could be expected to develop EXCEPT

(A) sustained rise in systemic blood pressure
(B) cardiomegaly and heart failure
(C) cerebral edema and seizures
(D) electrolyte abnormalities
(E) disseminated intravascular coagulation

30

88. A full-term infant is born after a normal pregnancy; delivery, however, is complicated by marginal placental separation. At 12 hours of age the child, although appearing to be in good health, passes a bloody meconium stool. For determining the etiology of the bleeding, which of the following diagnostic procedures should be performed first?

(A) A barium enema
(B) An Apt test
(C) Gastric lavage with normal saline
(D) An upper gastrointestinal series
(E) A platelet count, prothrombin time, and partial thromboplastin time

89. Which of the following patterns noted on continuous fetal heart rate monitoring warrants immediate delivery of the infant?

(A) Baseline variability with periodic acceleration
(B) Increasing baseline variability (saltatory pattern)
(C) Early deceleration pattern
(D) Late deceleration without baseline variability
(E) Variable deceleration with baseline variability

90. A healthy premature infant who weighs 950 g (2 lb, 1 1/2 oz) is fed undiluted breast milk to provide 120 cal/kg per day. Over ensuing weeks the baby is most apt to develop

(A) hypernatremia
(B) hypocalcemia
(C) blood in the stool
(D) metabolic acidosis
(E) vitamin E deficiency

91. An infant weighing 1400 g (3 lb) is born at 32 weeks gestation in a delivery room that has an ambient temperature of 24°C (75°F). Within a few minutes of birth, this infant is likely to exhibit all the following EXCEPT

(A) pallor
(B) shivering
(C) a fall in body temperature
(D) increased respiratory rate
(E) metabolic acidosis

92. A primiparous woman whose blood type is O-positive gives birth at term to an infant who has A-positive blood and a hematocrit of 55%. A serum bilirubin level obtained at 36 hours of age is 12 mg per 100 ml. Which of the following laboratory findings would be LEAST characteristic of ABO hemolytic disease?

(A) An elevated reticulocyte count
(B) A negative direct Coombs' test
(C) Fragmented red blood cells in the blood smear
(D) Nucleated red blood cells in the blood smear
(E) Spherocytes on blood smear

93. A 3-day-old infant born at 32 weeks gestation and weighing 1700 g (3 lb, 12 oz) has three episodes of apnea, each lasting 20 to 25 seconds and occurring after a feeding. During these episodes the heart rate drops from 140 to 100 beats per minute and the child remains motionless; between episodes, however, the child displays normal activity. Blood sugar is 50 mg per 100 ml and serum calcium is normal. The child's apneic periods most likely are

(A) due to an immature respiratory center
(B) a part of periodic breathing
(C) secondary to hypoglycemia
(D) manifestations of seizures
(E) evidence of underlying pulmonary disease

94. Two infants are born at 36 weeks gestation. Infant A weighs 2600 g (5 lb, 12 oz) and infant B weighs 1600 g (3 lb, 8 oz). Infant B is more likely to have all the following problems EXCEPT

(A) congenital malformations
(B) low hematocrit
(C) symptomatic hypoglycemia
(D) aspiration pneumonia
(E) future growth retardation

95. Which of the following statements characterizes the late anemia of prematurity?

(A) The platelet count is diminished
(B) The reticulocyte count is elevated
(C) It cannot occur in the presence of a normal serum tocopherol level
(D) It can be prevented by a diet high in polyunsaturated fatty acids
(E) Iron deficiency is present

96. The infant pictured below is 2 weeks old. He was delivered at term after a long and difficult labor. He weighed 4200 g (9 lb, 4 oz) at birth. The lesions shown on his arm and back are reddish-purple and indurated. Which of the following diagnoses is most likely to be correct?

(A) Erythema toxicum neonatorum
(B) Sclerema neonatorum
—(C) Subcutaneous fat necrosis
(D) Urticaria pigmentosa
(E) Mongolian spots

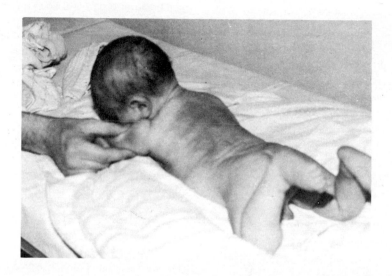

97. A 1-day-old infant who was born by a difficult forceps delivery is alert and active. However, she does not move her left arm, which she keeps internally rotated by her side with the forearm extended and pronated; she also does not move it during a Moro reflex. The rest of her physical examination is normal. This clinical picture most likely indicates

(A) fracture of the left clavicle
(B) fracture of the left humerus
—(C) left-sided Erb-Duchenne paralysis
(D) left-sided Klumpke's paralysis
(E) spinal injury with left hemiparesis

98. At 43 weeks gestation a long, thin infant is delivered who is apneic, limp, pale, and covered with "pea soup" amniotic fluid. The first step in the resuscitation of this infant after delivery should be

＼ (A) suction of the trachea under direct vision
(B) artificial ventilation with bag and mask
(C) artificial ventilation with endotracheal tube
(D) administration of 100% oxygen by mask
(E) catheterization of the umbilical vein

99. Which of the following statements about periventricular/subependymal hemorrhage in newborn infants is true?

(A) Clinical manifestations appear within minutes of a serious hypoxic episode
(B) It most commonly produces sudden severe neurologic deterioration
(C) It is seldom found in infants weighing less than 1500 g
(D) Systemic signs include an acute drop in hematocrit and arterial P_{O_2} and a marked fall in pH
(E) Posthemorrhagic ventricular dilatation cannot be evaluated adequately except by CAT scan

100. Initial examination of a full-term infant weighing less than 2500 g (5 lb, 8 oz) shows edema over the dorsum of her hands and feet. Which of the following findings would support a diagnosis of Turner's syndrome?

(A) A liver palpable to 2 cm below the costal margin
(B) Tremulous movements and ankle clonus
(C) Redundant skin folds at the nape of the neck
(D) A transient, longitudinal division of the body into a red half and a pale half
(E) Softness of the parietal bones at the vertex

101. After an uneventful labor and delivery, an infant is born at 32 weeks gestation weighing 1500 g (3 lb, 5 oz). Respiratory difficulty develops immediately after birth and increases in intensity thereafter. The child's mother (gravida 3, para 2, no abortions) previously lost an infant because of hyaline membrane disease. At 6 hours of age the child's respiratory rate is 60 per minute. Examination reveals grunting, intercostal retraction, nasal flaring, and marked cyanosis in room air. Physiologic abnormalities compatible with these data include

(A) decreased lung compliance, reduced lung volume, left-to-right shunt of blood
(B) decreased lung compliance, reduced lung volume, right-to-left shunt of blood
(C) decreased lung compliance, increased lung volume, left-to-right shunt of blood
(D) normal lung compliance, reduced lung volume, left-to-right shunt of blood
(E) normal lung compliance, increased lung volume, right-to-left shunt of blood

102. Shortly after birth, an infant develops abdominal distension and begins to drool. When she is given her first feeding, it runs out the side of her mouth and she coughs and chokes. Physical examination reveals tachypnea, intercostal retractions, and bilateral pulmonary rales. The esophageal anomaly that most commonly causes these signs and symptoms is illustrated by

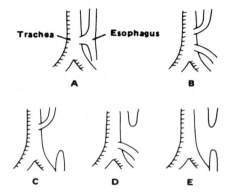

(A) figure A
(B) figure B
(C) figure C
 (D) figure D
(E) figure E

103. Failure to administer vitamin K prophylactically to a newborn infant is associated with which of the following?

(A) A deficiency of factor V
—(B) A prolonged prothrombin time
(C) Development of hemorrhagic manifestations within 24 hours of delivery
(D) Manifestations that are more severe in male than female infants
(E) A greater likelihood of developing symptoms if the infant is fed cow's milk rather than breast milk

104. Which of the following drugs given during the last 2 weeks of pregnancy is the most likely to have deleterious effects on the fetus?

—(A) Propranolol
(B) Penicillin
(C) Aluminum hydroxide
(D) Hydantoin
(E) Heparin

105. At the time of delivery, a woman is noted to have a large volume of amniotic fluid. At 6 hours of age her baby begins regurgitating small amounts of mucus and bile-stained fluid. Physical examination of the infant is normal, and an abdominal x-ray is obtained (shown below). The most likely diagnosis of this infant's disorder is

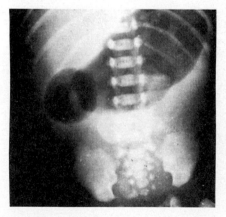

(A) gastric duplication
(B) pyloric stenosis
(C) esophageal atresia
— (D) duodenal atresia
(E) midgut volvulus

106. Which of the following statements about the infant pictured below is true?

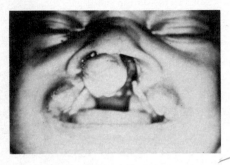

(A) Parenteral alimentation is recommended to prevent aspiration
(B) Surgical closure of the palatal defect should be done before 3 months of age
(C) Good anatomic closure will preclude the development of speech defects
— (D) Recurrent otitis media and hearing loss are likely complications
(E) The chance that a sibling also would be affected is 1 in 1000

107. A woman (gravida 3, para 0, 2 abortions) who is in early labor comes to her community hospital at 28 weeks gestation. The hospital, which has an excellent obstetric service but no intensive-care nursery, is located 25 miles from the nearest referral perinatal center. To maximize the child's chances for survival without causing unnecessary hardship to the woman, which of the following courses of action would be most advisable?

(A) Transfer the woman immediately to the referral perinatal center
(B) Transfer the infant to the referral perinatal center immediately after birth
(C) Transfer the infant to the referral perinatal center at the first sign of illness
(D) Transfer the infant to the referral perinatal center only if a severe illness develops
(E) Keep the woman and her infant at the community hospital

108. The chance of severe hypoglycemia in the infant of a diabetic mother can be lessened by all the following EXCEPT

(A) careful control of the maternal blood glucose levels during pregnancy
— (B) maternal intravenous loading with 10% glucose beginning 2 to 4 hours prior to the expected time of delivery
(C) careful glucose monitoring of the infant
(D) early feedings of the infant
(E) maintenance of the infant in a neutral thermal environment

DIRECTIONS: Each question below contains four suggested responses of which
one or more is correct. Select

A	if	**1, 2, and 3**	are correct
B	if	**1 and 3**	are correct
C	if	**2 and 4**	are correct
D	if	**4**	is correct
E	if	**1, 2, 3, and 4**	are correct

109. In the management of an infant who has hyperbilirubinemia, factors to be considered in assessing the risk of kernicterus include the presence of

(1) acidosis
(2) hypoxia
(3) hypoalbuminemia
(4) cold stress

110. Normal full-term newborn infants can demonstrate which of the following reflex reactions?

(1) Stepping reflex
(2) Palmar grasp
(3) Placing reflex
(4) Parachute reaction

111. An infant born to a heroin addict who has received no prenatal care is likely to exhibit

(1) prematurity and low birth weight
(2) onset of withdrawal symptoms within the first 2 days of life
(3) hyperirritability and coarse tremors
(4) vomiting and diarrhea

112. The diagnosis of meconium ileus in a neonate who has signs of intestinal obstruction is supported by

(1) a family history of cystic fibrosis
(2) palpation of several doughy masses throughout the abdomen
(3) the radiographic presence of unevenly dilated, granular-looking loops of bowel
(4) a greenish discoloration of the abdominal wall

113. A previously healthy full-term infant has several episodes of duskiness and apnea during the second day of life. Diagnostic considerations should include

(1) bacterial meningitis
(2) congenital heart disease
(3) seizure disorder
(4) hypoglycemia

114. A woman gives birth to twins at
38 weeks gestation. The first twin
weighs 2800 g (6 lb, 3 oz) and has a
hematocrit of 70%; the second twin
weighs 2100 g (4 lb, 10 oz) and has a
hematocrit of 40%. Correct statements
concerning these infants include which
of the following?

(1) The first twin is at risk for devel-
     oping respiratory distress, cy-
     anosis, and congestive heart failure
(2) The first twin may have hyperbili-
     rubinemia and convulsions
(3) The second twin may be pale,
     tachycardic, and hypotensive
(4) The second twin probably has hy-
     dramnios of the amniotic sac

DIRECTIONS: Each group of questions below consists of lettered headings followed by a set of numbered items. For each numbered item select the **one** lettered heading with which it is **most** closely associated. Each lettered heading may be used **once, more than once, or not at all.**

Questions 115–118

For each description of congenital anomalies that follows, select the major abnormality with which it is most likely to be associated.

(A) Deafness
(B) Seizures
(C) Wilms' tumor
(D) Congestive heart failure
(E) Optic glioma

115. Nonfamilial bilateral absence of the iris (aniridia)

116. Heterochromia of the iris, broad nasal root, fusion of the eyebrows, and white forelock

117. Flat capillary hemangioma over the anterior scalp and one side of the face

118. Hypopigmented oval macules on the skin of the trunk and extremities

Questions 119–122

For each jaundiced infant described below, select the lettered curve on the graph that best represents the expected course of that infant's serum bilirubin.

119. A premature neonate who is otherwise normal

120. A full-term neonate who is found to have septicemia on day 4

121. A full-term neonate with hypothyroidism

122. A full-term neonate who has erythroblastosis fetalis

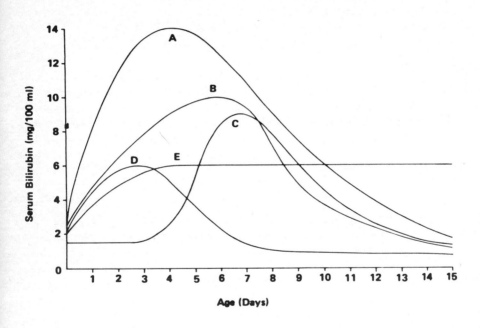

The Newborn Infant

Answers

83. The answer is D. *(Forbes, ed 2. pp 1-15.)* The administration of radioactive isotopes to the mother is a recognized contraindication to breast feeding. A healthy infant may be fed as early as 12 hours after cesarean delivery. The mother is usually most comfortable in a reclining position in bed with the infant supported by pillows. Low-birth-weight and hospitalized infants can be fed breast milk either directly or from storage after heating or freezing.

84. The answer is A. *(Forbes, ed 2. p 25.)* Iron, linoleic acid, and vitamin C are not provided in adequate amounts for an infant by a diet of whole cow's milk and therefore need to be added to the diet as a supplement. Whole cow's milk is very high in protein, which leads to its high renal solute load. Infants fed on whole cow's milk should have supplementation of their diet with water, particularly when it is hot or if they have diarrhea.

85. The answer is C. *(Behrman, ed 12. p 1011.)* It is important to make the diagnosis of choanal atresia quickly in that it responds to treatment but may be lethal if unrecognized and untreated. Most neonates are obligate nose breathers since they cannot breathe adequately through their mouths. Infants with choanal atresia have increased breathing difficulty during feeding and sleeping and improve when crying. A variety of temporizing measures to maintain an open airway have been used, including oropharyngeal airways, positioning, tongue fixation, and endotracheal intubation, but surgical correction with placement of nasal tubes is effective.

86. The answer is B. *(Finberg, p 18.)* A normal 2-week-old infant has a basal caloric expenditure of about 65 cal/kg per day. Adding calories for activity and growth brings the caloric requirement to about 110 cal/kg. A 3.5-kg infant, therefore, requires about 385 cal in the diet per day. Standard infant formulas have a caloric density of 0.67 cal/ml, so it would take about 575 ml of infant formula per day to supply adequate calories for this infant. For the infant in question, 60 ml four times a day (240 ml per day) is less than half of the amount that the infant needs and should be of concern. The other factors in the question are normal for the infant's age.

87. The answer is A. *(Avery, ed 2. pp 183–188. Fanaroff, ed 3. pp 191–192.)* During a period of asphyxia, hypoxemia and acidosis and poor perfusion can damage a neonate's brain, heart, kidney, liver, and lungs. The resulting clinical abnormalities include cerebral edema, irritability, seizures, cardiomegaly, heart failure, renal failure, poor liver function, and respiratory distress syndrome. There may be excessively high pulmonary arterial pressure, resulting in a persistent right-to-left shunt across a patent ductus arteriosus or foramen ovale.

88. The answer is B. *(Avery and Taeusch, ed 5. pp 316–317.)* Hematemesis and melena are not uncommon in the neonatal period, especially if gross placental bleeding has occurred at the time of delivery. The diagnostic procedure that should be done first is the Apt test, which differentiates fetal from adult hemoglobin in a bloody specimen. If the blood in an affected infant's gastric contents or stool is maternal in origin, further workup of the infant is obviated.

89. The answer is D. *(Fanaroff, ed 3. pp 95–107.)* Baseline variability with or without periodic acceleration of the fetal heart rate is a sign of fetal well-being. Increasing baseline variability (saltatory pattern) may represent early compromise of fetal oxygenation. The early deceleration pattern is due to pressure of the anterior fontanel on the cervix and is not a sign of fetal distress. The variable deceleration pattern indicates umbilical cord compression. The late deceleration pattern signifies fetal hypoxemia. Both of these last two patterns in association with loss of baseline variability are signs of severe fetal compromise and warrant immediate delivery of the infant.

90. The answer is B. *(Fanaroff, ed 3. pp 302–307.)* The average healthy low-birth-weight infant of this size requires a daily intake of 100 to 150 mg/kg of calcium. It is usually impossible with any combination of parenteral and enteral nutrition to match what the infant would have accumulated in utero. Breast milk has less calcium (and phosphorus) than commercial formulas. One may supplement the breast milk with calcium or mix it with commercial formulas designed for the premature infant.

91. The answer is B. *(Avery, ed 2. pp 171–181.)* A room temperature of 24°C (approximately 75°F) provides a cold environment for preterm infants weighing less than 1500 g (3 lb, 4 oz). Aside from the fact that these infants emerge from a warm 37.6°C (99.5°F) intrauterine environment, at birth they are wet, have a relatively large surface area for their weight, and have little subcutaneous fat. Within minutes of delivery the infants are likely to become pale or blue and their body temperatures will drop. In order to bring body temperature back to normal they must increase their metabolic rate; ventilation, in turn, must increase proportionally to ensure an adequate oxygen supply. Because a preterm infant is likely to have respiratory problems and be unable to oxygenate adequately, lactate can accumulate and lead to a metabolic acidosis. Infants rarely shiver in response to a need to increase heat production.

92. The answer is B. *(Behrman, ed 12. p 388.)* If a mother is O-positive and her baby is A-positive, the baby has a 10-percent chance of developing hemolytic disease. Hemolytic disease and jaundice caused by a major blood-group incompatibility are usually less severe than with Rh incompatibility. Although the hematocrit of affected infants usually is normal, elevation of the reticulocyte count and the presence of nucleated red blood cells and spherocytes in the blood smear provide evidence of hemolysis. In comparison with hemolytic disease caused by Rh incompatibility, where it is usually strongly positive, major blood-group incompatibility is associated with a direct Coombs' test that is most frequently weakly positive.

93. The answer is A. *(Fanaroff, ed 3. pp 456–460.)* Apneic spells are characterized by an absence of respirations for more than 20 seconds or by bradycardia and cyanosis (or by both). Periods of apnea are thought to be secondary to an incompletely developed respiratory center and are associated most commonly with prematurity. Although seizures, hypoglycemia, and pulmonary disease accompanied by hypoxia all can lead to apnea, these etiologies are unlikely in the infant described, given that no unusual movements occur during the apneic spells, that the blood sugar level is more than 40 mg per 100 ml, and that the child appears well between spells. Periodic breathing, a common pattern of respiration in low-birth-weight babies, is characterized by periods of rapid respiration, lasting 10 to 15 seconds, that alternate with periods of apnea, lasting 5 to 10 seconds.

94. The answer is B. *(Fanaroff, ed 3. pp 70–78.)* Small-for-dates infants are subject to a different set of complications than preterm infants whose size is appropriate for gestational age. The small-for-dates infants have a higher incidence of major congenital anomalies and are at increased risk for future growth retardation, especially if length and head circumference as well as weight are small for gestational age. They also are at a greater risk for neonatal asphyxia and the meconium aspiration syndrome, which can lead to pneumothorax, pneumomediastinum, or pulmonary hemorrhage. These, rather than hyaline membrane disease, are the major pulmonary problems in these infants. Because neonatal symptomatic hypoglycemia is commonly found in small-for-dates infants, careful blood glucose monitoring and early feeding are appropriate precautions. Elevated hematocrit is common in these infants.

95. The answer is E. *(Avery, ed 2. pp 237–239.)* The late anemia of prematurity results from iron deficiency. The premature infant's iron stores depend upon the total body hemoglobin at birth. This is influenced by the infant's size and the circumstances of delivery. The amount of blood withdrawn for laboratory studies and the amount, if any, transfused will affect the timing and the extent of the problem. Iron should be begun when the infant has obtained a weight one and a half times that of birth weight.

96. The answer is C. *(Behrman, ed 12. pp 1705–1706.)* Subcutaneous fat necrosis is found in large infants who suffer a long or difficult labor and delivery. Lesions usually appear at about 1 week of age over cheeks and extensor surfaces. They vary in size, may be colorless or reddish-purple, and feel firm with a sharp border. They usually produce no symptoms and regress gradually over a period of weeks. Hypercalcemia may be present. The other diagnoses listed in the question would be suggested by very different appearances.

97. The answer is C. *(Behrman, ed 12. pp 359–360.)* In a difficult delivery in which traction is applied to the head and neck, several injuries, including all those listed in the question, may occur. Erb-Duchenne paralysis affects the fifth and sixth cervical nerves; the affected arm cannot be abducted or externally rotated at the shoulder, and the forearm cannot be supinated. Injury to the seventh and eighth cervical and first thoracic nerves (Klumpke's paralysis) results in palsy of the hand and also can produce Horner's syndrome. Fractures in the upper limb are not associated with a characteristic posture, and passive movement usually elicits pain. Spinal injury causes complete paralysis below the level of injury.

98. The answer is A. *(Avery and Taeusch, ed 5. pp 107–108.)* Infants who are postmature (more than 42 weeks gestation) and show evidence of chronic placental insufficiency (low birth weight for gestational age and wasted appearance) have a higher than average chance of being asphyxiated, and passage of meconium into the amniotic fluid thus places these infants at risk for meconium aspiration. To prevent or minimize this risk, these infants should have immediate nasopharyngeal suction as their heads are delivered. Immediately after delivery and before initiation of respiration their tracheas should be carefully and thoroughly suctioned through an endotracheal tube under direct vision with a laryngoscope. Afterwards, appropriate resuscitative measures should be undertaken to establish adequate ventilation and circulation. Artificial ventilation performed before tracheal suction could force meconium into smaller airways.

99. The answer is D. *(Fanaroff, ed 3. pp 367–369.)* Periventricular/subependymal hemorrhage is the most common type of intracranial hemorrhage in newborn infants. It occurs in approximately 45 percent of premature infants weighing less than 1500 g. Clinical manifestations may occur 24 to 28 hours after a serious hypoxic episode. This type of hemorrhage is not usually catastrophic, and it commonly produces only subtle neurologic deterioration. There may be an acute drop in hematocrit and arterial P_{O_2} and a marked metabolic acidosis. Serial ultrasound examination of the ventricles and brain are required for diagnosis and proper follow-up.

100. The answer is C. *(Behrman, ed 12. pp 331–335, 1502.)* Turner's syndrome is a genetic disorder characterized by a 45,XO karyotype. At birth affected infants have low weights, short stature, edema over the dorsum of the hands and feet, and loose skin folds at the nape of the neck. Coarse tremulous movements accompanied by ankle clonus; vascular instability as evidenced, for example, by a harlequin color change (a transient, longitudinal division of a body into red and pale halves); softness of parietal bones at the vertex (craniotabes); and a liver that is palpable down to 2 cm below the costal margin are all findings often demonstrated by normal infants and are of no diagnostic significance in the clinical situation presented.

101. The answer is B. *(Fanaroff, ed 3. pp 427–428.)* For the child described in the question, prematurity and the clinical picture presented make the diagnosis of hyaline membrane disease likely. In this disease lung compliance can be reduced to 10 to 20 percent of normal; lung volume also is reduced and there may be a 30- to 60-percent right-to-left shunt of blood. Some of the shunt may result from a patent ductus arteriosus or foramen ovale, and some may be due to shunting in the lung. Minute ventilation is higher than normal and affected infants must work harder in order to sustain adequate breathing.

102. The answer is D. *(Behrman, ed 12. pp 893–894.)* Abdominal distension, choking, drooling, and coughing associated with feedings are symptoms of esophageal anomalies. The anomaly illustrated by figure D is the most common; that of figure A may be diagnosed after repeated episodes of pneumonia. The anomalies in figures E and C are associated with all the same symptoms except abdominal distension, which cannot develop because air cannot enter the gastrointestinal tract. B and C are the least common; in these the upper esophageal segment is connected directly to the trachea and massive entry of fluid into the lungs occurs.

103. The answer is B. *(Behrman, ed 12. p 1247.)* Failure to give vitamin K prophylactically to newborn infants is associated with a decline in the levels of vitamin K-dependent coagulation factors. In less than 1 percent of infants (but especially those fed human breast milk), the levels reached are low enough to produce hemorrhagic manifestations on the second or third day of life. These manifestations include melena, hematuria, and bleeding from the navel; intracranial hemorrhage and hypovolemic shock are serious complications. Diagnosis of this condition is indicated by a prolonged prothrombin time, which reflects inadequate concentrations of factors II, VII, and X.

104. The answer is A. *(Fanaroff, ed 3. pp 154–156.)* The effect of a drug on the fetus is determined by the nature of the drug and by the timing and degree of exposure. Heparin does not cross the placental barrier and cannot directly affect the fetus once pregnancy is well established. Hydantoin may cause birth defects when given during the first trimester. Penicillin and aluminum hydroxide have not been found to affect the fetus. Propranolol, which may cause growth retardation when given throughout pregnancy, diminishes the ability of an asphyxiated infant to increase heart rate and cardiac output. It has also been associated with hypoglycemia.

105. The answer is D. *(Avery, ed 2. pp 812–813.)* The finding of hydramnios signals high intestinal obstruction, signs of which include abdominal distension and early and repeated regurgitation. Distension may not be present if the obstruction is very high or if vomiting keeps the intestine decompressed. The bile-stained vomitus of the infant places the obstruction distal to the ampulla of Vater, eliminating esophageal atresia and pyloric stenosis from consideration. The "double bubble" sign on the x-ray is characteristic of duodenal atresia, which is compatible with the history. Midgut volvulus, which may obstruct the bowel in the area of the duodenojejunal junction, most often produces signs after an affected infant is 3 or 4 days old, and several loops of small bowel are typically seen on x-ray. Gastric duplication does not usually produce intestinal obstruction; a cystic mass may be palpated on abdominal examination.

106. The answer is D. *(Behrman, ed 12. pp 881–882.)* The infant pictured has bilateral cleft lip and palate. This defect occurs in 4 to 7 percent of the siblings of affected infants; its incidence in the general population, is 1 in 1000. Although affected infants are likely to have feeding problems initially, these problems usually can be overcome by feeding in a propped-up position and using special nipples. Complications include recurrent otitis media and hearing loss as well as speech defects, which may be present in spite of good anatomic closure. Repair of a cleft lip usually is performed within the first 2 months of life; the palate is repaired later, usually between the ages of 6 months and 5 years.

107. The answer is A. *(AAP-ACOG, p 187.)* The pregnancy of the woman described in the question is considered high-risk by virtue of her history of abortions and the premature onset of labor. The woman's infant will very likely require neonatal intensive care. Statistics show that the mortality for low-birth-weight infants is lowest if they are born in centers having facilities for prenatal intensive care (one third of all deaths of premature infants occur within 24 hours of birth). For this reason, and because a mother's womb is thought to be the best "transport incubator" available, the woman described should be transferred to the referral perinatal center immediately (i.e., before the birth of her child).

108. The answer is B. *(Avery, ed 2. pp 295–297.)* Glucose loading of the mother will result in fetal hyperglycemia, which causes insulin release and reactive hypoglycemia. Careful medical support of the antepartum woman diminishes the hypertrophy of the fetal islet cells. Careful monitoring of the infant with early feeding or intravenous infusion of glucose can prevent hypoglycemia. A neutral thermal environment diminishes glucose consumption and, therefore, helps with glucose homeostasis.

109. The answer is E (all). *(Fanaroff, ed 3. pp 764–765.)* Factors that reduce the amount of unconjugated bilirubin bound to albumin (and therefore cause an increase in free unconjugated bilirubin) increase the risk of kernicterus. Among these factors are the following: hypoalbuminemia; acidosis, which decreases the affinity of bilirubin for albumin; and certain drugs (e.g., salicylates and sulfonamides) and other compounds (such as nonesterified fatty acids, which are elevated during cold stress) that compete with bilirubin for albumin binding sites. Acidosis and hypoxia also are believed to increase brain-cell susceptibility to bilirubin toxicity.

110. The answer is A (1,2,3). *(Avery and Taeusch, ed 5. pp 654–655.)* Normal term neonates demonstrate a large number of reflex patterns that are mediated by the brainstem or spinal cord. These reactions include the Moro (startle) reflex; the sucking and rooting reflexes; the stepping reflex, by which movements of forward progression are elicited on a flat surface; the placing reflex, which produces leg flexion; and the palmar and plantar grasps, which are induced by slight pressure on the palms and soles. The parachute reaction, which is extension of the arms and hands that occurs when an infant in the prone position is brought sharply toward a firm surface, does not appear until the age of 9 months.

111. The answer is E (all). *(Behrman, ed 12. pp 394–395.)* Infants born to narcotic addicts are morely likely than other children to exhibit a variety of problems, including perinatal complications, prematurity, and low birth weight. The onset of withdrawal commonly occurs during an infant's first 2 days of life and is characterized by hyperirritability and coarse tremors, along with vomiting, diarrhea, fever, high-pitched cry, and hyperventilation; seizures and respiratory depression are less common.

112. The answer is A (1,2,3). *(Behrman, ed 12. pp 377–378.)* Meconium ileus occurs in newborn infants who have cystic fibrosis, because the paucity of normal pancreatic enzymes makes their meconium abnormally tenacious. Affected neonates present with signs of intestinal obstruction, and doughy masses of intestine are palpable throughout the abdomen; no discoloration of the abdominal wall occurs. Plain films of the abdomen characteristically show unevenly dilated loops of bowel that, because of a mixture of meconium and air, appear granular.

113. The answer is E (all). *(Fanaroff, ed 3. pp 562–563.)* Apnea is common in premature infants but is distinctly unusual in the term baby. When it occurs there is almost always an identifiable cause. Sepsis, congenital heart disease, seizures, and hypoglycemia are recognized causes of apnea in term newborns.

114. The answer is A (1,2,3). *(Fanaroff, ed 3. p 714.)* Twin-to-twin transfusions occur in about 15 percent of monochorionic twins and commonly cause intrauterine death. This disorder should be suspected when the hematocrits of twins differ by more than 15. The donor twin is likely to have oligohydramnios, anemia, and hypovolemia with evidence of shock; the recipient twin is likely to have hydramnios and plethora and to be larger than the donor twin. As the central venous hematocrit rises above 65%, infants may develop hyperviscosity, respiratory distress, hyperbilirubinemia, hypoglycemia, hypocalcemia, renal vein thrombosis, congestive heart failure, and convulsions.

115–118. The answers are: 115-C, 116-A, 117-B, 118-B. *(Smith, ed 3. pp 182–183.)* Sporadic aniridia is found in 1 to 2 percent of children with Wilm's tumor. Genitourinary anomalies and hemihypertrophy are associated with this tumor in 13 percent of patients.

Waardenburg's syndrome is inherited as an autosomal dominant trait with variable penetrance. It includes, in decreasing order of frequency, the following anomalies: lateral displacement of the medial canthi; broad nasal bridge; medial hyperplasia of the eyebrows; partial albinism commonly expressed by a white forelock or heterochromia (or both); and deafness in 20 percent of cases.

A flat capillary hemangioma in the distribution of the trigeminal nerve is the basic lesion in the Sturge-Weber syndrome. The malformation also involves the meninges and results in anoxic damage to the underlying cerebral cortex. The damage is manifested clinically by grand mal seizures, mental deficiency, and hemiparesis or hemianopia on the contralateral side. The etiology is unknown.

Infants who have tuberous sclerosis often are born with hypopigmented oval or irregularly shaped skin macules. Cerebral sclerotic tubers are also present from birth and become visible radiographically during the second year of life. Myoclonic seizures, present in infancy, may convert to grand mal seizures later in childhood. Adenoma sebaceum appears at 2 to 5 years of age. The disease, which also affects the eyes, kidneys, heart, bones, and lungs, is inherited as an autosomal dominant trait with variable expression; new mutations are very common.

119–122. The answers are: 119-B, 120-C, 121-E, 122-A. *(Behrman, ed 12. pp 378–381.)* In premature infants who have physiologic jaundice (curve B), serum bilirubin levels usually peak at 8 to 12 mg per 100 ml at 5 to 7 days of age; jaundice disappears after the tenth day of life. Physiologic jaundice in full-term neonates (curve D), on the other hand, usually appears at 2 to 3 days of age; peak bilirubin levels of about 5 to 6 mg per 100 ml may appear at 2 to 4 days of age. Bilirubin levels drop below 2 mg per 100 ml within a few days.

Jaundice in infants who have hypothyroidism (curve E) may initially appear to be physiologic. However, jaundice in these infants (as well as infants who have pyloric stenosis) can persist for several weeks.

In neonates born with erythroblastosis fetalis (curve A), jaundice is apparent in the first 24 hours of life. Bilirubin accumulates rapidly, reaching a peak level that varies with the degree of hemolysis and hepatic function. The duration of jaundice is dependent on the severity of the disease.

Curve C on the graph is compatible with a diagnosis of septicemia. In this disorder jaundice usually appears between the fourth and seventh days of life; as the infection responds to treatment, the bilirubin levels return to normal.

The Cardiovascular System

DIRECTIONS: Each question below contains five suggested responses. Select the **one best** response to each question.

123. In an infant an important noncardiac manifestation of digitalis toxicity is

(A) fever
(B) dizziness
(C) vomiting
(D) visual disturbances
(E) urticaria

124. A 15-year-old girl with short stature who has neck webbing and sexual infantilism is found to have coarctation of the aorta. The most likely diagnosis is

(A) Marfan's syndrome
(B) Down's syndrome
(C) Turner's syndrome
(D) Ellis–van Creveld syndrome
(E) an unrelated group of findings

125. Electrocardiography of a cyanotic 2-day-old infant suggests right ventricular enlargement. The chest x-ray is presented below. The most likely diagnosis is

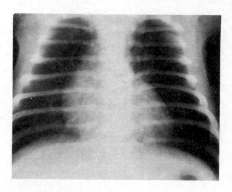

(A) tetralogy of Fallot
(B) transposition of the great vessels
(C) tricuspid atresia
(D) pulmonic valve atresia
(E) Ebstein's anomaly

126. The incidence of congenital heart disease in the offspring of mothers with congenital heart disease is

(A) 1 percent
(B) 3 percent
(C) 8 percent
—(D) 14 percent
(E) 23 percent

127. A male infant presents at age 2 days with a harsh grade 3/6 pansystolic murmur in the third and fourth spaces along the left sternal border with radiation to the apex. The murmur sounds louder by one grade the next day and is associated with a thrill. The findings remain unchanged until day four when he develops a diastolic grade II/VI rumble over the apex in addition to the pansystolic murmur and thrill. These findings point to a diagnosis of

— (A) ventricular septal defect
(B) ventricular septal defect and aortic regurgitation
(C) atrial septal defect
(D) atrial septal defect and pulmonary regurgitation
(E) none of the above

128. Pulmonary vascular resistance in an infant begins to diminish rapidly following delivery. This physiologic change is thought to be regulated primarily by

— (A) a rise in arterial P_{O_2}
(B) a decrease in intrathoracic pressure
(C) a reduction in the tortuosity of the pulmonary vasculature
(D) closure of the ductus arteriosus
(E) release of humoral factors after cessation of placental circulation

129. A 2-year-old boy is brought into the emergency room with a complaint of fever for 6 days and development of a limp. On examination he is found to have an erythematous macular exanthem over his body, ocular conjunctivitis, dry, cracked lips, a red throat, and cervical lymphadenopathy. The skin around his nails is peeling. There is a grade II/VI vibratory systolic ejection murmur at the lower left sternal border. He refuses to bear weight on his left leg. A white blood cell count and differential show predominantly neutrophils with increased platelets on smear. The most likely diagnosis is

(A) scarlet fever
(B) rheumatic fever
—(C) Kawasaki disease
(D) juvenile rheumatoid arthritis
(E) infectious mononucleosis

130. An ill-appearing 2-week-old girl is brought to the emergency room. She is pale and dyspneic with a respiratory rate of 80 per minute. Heart rate is 195 per minute, sounds are distant, and there is a suggestion of a gallop. There is cardiomegaly by x-ray. An echocardiogram demonstrates poor ventricular function, dilated ventricles, and dilation of the left atrium. Electrocardiogram shows ventricular depolarization complexes that have low voltage. The diagnosis suggested by this clinical picture is

(A) myocarditis
(B) endocardial fibroelastosis
(C) pericarditis
(D) aberrant left coronary artery arising from pulmonary artery
(E) glycogen storage disease of the heart

131. Individuals who have chronic hypoxia have an increased hematocrit. The stimulation of red blood cell production has been attributed to release of erythropoietin by the

(A) spleen
(B) liver
(C) kidneys
(D) bone marrow
(E) lungs

132. A newborn infant has mild cyanosis, diaphoresis, poor peripheral pulses, hepatomegaly, and cardiomegaly. Respiratory rate is 60 per minute, and heart rate is 230 per minute. The child most likely has congestive heart failure caused by

(A) a large atrial septal defect and valvular pulmonic stenosis
(B) a ventricular septal defect and transposition of the great vessels
(C) atrial flutter and partial atrioventricular block
(D) hypoplastic left heart syndrome
(E) paroxysmal atrial tachycardia

133. A 3-year-old child has had two episodes of syncope. On examination, blood pressure is normal in the arms and legs; no murmurs are heard. Prior neurologic evaluation revealed no neurologic abnormalities. The study most likely to aid in diagnosing this child's condition would be

(A) electrocardiography
(B) vectorcardiography
(C) echocardiography
(D) isotope angiography
(E) cardiac catheterization

134. A 5-year-old boy presents with a grade V/VI harsh ejection systolic murmur in the second interspace at the right sternal border. The murmur radiates to the neck and upper left sternal border. The right brachial pulse is brisk, the left diminished. Blood pressures are right arm 110/60 mmHg, left arm 100/60 mmHg. He has a small chin, full lips, open mouth, upturned nose, and wide-set eyes. An electrocardiogram shows left ventricular hypertrophy. The most likely defect would be

(A) bicuspid aortic valve
(B) valvular aortic stenosis
(C) discrete subvalvular aortic stenosis
(D) supravalvular aortic stenosis
(E) aortic coarctation

135. Congestive heart failure from congenital heart disease is encountered most frequently in which of the following age groups?

(A) Less than 6 months of age
(B) 6 to 12 months of age
(C) 1 to 5 years of age
(D) 6 to 15 years of age
(E) 16 to 21 years of age

136. A child with an atrial septal defect has an accentuated pulmonic closure sound; electrocardiography shows right ventricular hypertrophy. These findings suggest that the child most likely has

(A) valvular pulmonic stenosis
(B) infundibular pulmonic stenosis
(C) pulmonary hypertension
(D) congestive heart failure
(E) pulmonic regurgitation

137. A 2-year-old child with minimal cyanosis has a quadruple rhythm, a systolic murmur in the pulmonic area, and a middiastolic murmur along the lower left sternal border. An electrocardiogram is obtained and shows P pulmonale and a ventricular block pattern in the right chest leads. The child most likely has

(A) tricuspid regurgitation and pulmonic stenosis
(B) pulmonic stenosis and a ventricular septal defect (tetralogy of Fallot)
(C) an atrioventricular canal
(D) Ebstein's anomaly
(E) Wolff-Parkinson-White syndrome

138. A 4-year-old girl is brought to the pediatrician's office. Her father reports that she suddenly became pale and stopped running while he had been playfully chasing her. During play she had been very excited, laughing to the point at which "she almost lost her breath." After 30 minutes, she was no longer pale and wanted to resume the game. She has never had a previous episode nor ever been cyanotic. Her physical examination was normal as were her chest x-ray and echocardiogram. An electrocardiogram showed the pattern seen in the figure below, which shows

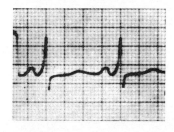

(A) paroxysmal ventricular tachycardia
(B) paroxysmal supraventricular tachycardia
(C) Wolff-Parkinson-White syndrome
(D) Stokes-Adams pattern
(E) excessive stress during play

139. Examination of a newborn infant reveals a heart rate of 60 beats per minute. At no time during the next 3 days does the rate rise above 68 beats per minute. Electrocardiography would be most likely to demonstrate

(A) second-degree atrioventricular block
(B) complete atrioventricular block
(C) complete atrioventricular block and atrial fibrillation
(D) sinus arrest with an idioventricular rhythm
(E) sinus bradycardia

140. A child has a history of spiking fevers, which have been as high as 40°C (104°F). She has spindle-shaped swelling of finger joints and complains of upper sternal pain. The most likely diagnosis is

(A) rheumatic fever
(B) juvenile rheumatoid arthritis
(C) toxic synovitis
(D) septic arthritis
(E) osteoarthritis

141. A 3-day-old infant has had progressive deepening cyanosis since birth but no respiratory distress. Chest radiography demonstrates no cardiomegaly and normal pulmonary vasculature. An electrocardiogram shows an axis of 120 degrees and right ventricular prominence. The congenital cardiac malformation most likely responsible for the cyanosis is

(A) tetralogy of Fallot
(B) transposition of the great vessels
(C) tricuspid atresia
(D) pulmonary atresia with intact ventricular septum
(E) total anomalous pulmonary venous return below the diaphragm

142. The presence of an endocardial cushion defect is associated with

(A) Turner's syndrome
(B) Noonan's syndrome
(C) Down's syndrome
(D) Marfan's syndrome
(E) Hunter-Hurler syndrome

DIRECTIONS: Each question below contains four suggested responses of which **one or more** is correct. Select

A	if	**1, 2, and 3**	are correct
B	if	**1 and 3**	are correct
C	if	**2 and 4**	are correct
D	if	**4**	is correct
E	if	**1, 2, 3, and 4**	are correct

143. A newborn infant who is in respiratory distress because of congestive heart failure would be likely to exhibit which of the following?

(1) Tachypnea
(2) Grunting
(3) Hyperpnea
(4) Periodic breathing

144. The hypoplastic left-heart syndrome describes a group of lesions that includes

(1) aortic atresia
(2) hypoplasia of the aortic arch
(3) mitral atresia
(4) endocardial fibroelastosis

145. A newborn infant weighing 2000 g (4 lb, 6 oz) presents with cyanosis; there is no evidence of respiratory distress. Cardiac catheterization reveals pulmonic valve atresia and pulmonary flow that derives from the aorta through a patent ductus arteriosus. Maintenance of adequate pulmonary blood flow may be achieved by

(1) aorticopulmonary anastomosis
(2) administration of E-type prostaglandins
(3) formalin infiltration of the ductus arteriosus
(4) pulmonary valvotomy

146. At birth the transition from fetal circulation is associated with a rapid decrease in pulmonary arterial resistance caused by

(1) increased oxygen tension producing pulmonary arterial vasodilation
(2) increased oxygen tension stimulating closure of the ductus arteriosus
(3) initial inspiration producing inflation of the lungs
(4) closure of the foramen ovale, producing increased right heart and, therefore, pulmonary arterial blood volume

147. A newborn infant of a diabetic mother presents with signs of congestive heart failure. Laboratory analysis is likely to reveal

(1) hypoglycemia
(2) hyperbilirubinemia
(3) hypocalcemia
(4) hyperinsulinemia

148. Which of the following manifestations of acute rheumatic fever can be relieved by salicylate or steroid therapy?

(1) Carditis
(2) Abdominal pain
(3) Arthritis
(4) Chorea

SUMMARY OF DIRECTIONS

A	B	C	D	E
1,2,3	1,3	2,4	4	All are
only	only	only	only	correct

149. An 8-year-old boy is brought into the hospital with a complaint of a seizure that occurred while chasing a friend. There is a history of recent onset of fatigue and heavier breathing than peers during play. On examination he is thin, in no distress, and without cyanosis, clubbing, edema, thrills, or murmurs. The pulmonic second sound is mildly accentuated. Neurologic examination reveals no abnormalities except for a mild hearing deficit. Further evaluation should be directed toward ruling out the possibility of

(1) long Q-T syndrome
(2) aortic stenosis
(3) primary pulmonary hypertension
(4) paroxysmal atrial tachycardia

150. A cyanotic 20-month-old child has a continuous murmur over the precordium and over the back. The child is in no visible distress. This clinical picture can be associated with which of the following disorders?

(1) Truncus arteriosus
(2) Total anomalous pulmonary venous return
(3) Tetralogy of Fallot
(4) Patent ductus arteriosus

151. The performance of an atrial septostomy during cardiac catheterization may be helpful in patients with which of the following?

(1) Tricuspid atresia with hypoplastic right ventricle
(2) Tricuspid atresia with ventricular septal defect
(3) Tricuspid atresia with severe pulmonic stenosis
(4) Tricuspid atresia with transposition of the great arteries

152. Cardiac catheterization shows that a child has a partial anomalous pulmonary venous return to the right atrium with an intact atrial septum. Pulmonary artery and right ventricular pressures are not elevated. Physical examination might be expected to reveal

(1) pulmonic ejection systolic murmur
(2) fixed wide splitting of the second heart sound
(3) right ventricular heave
(4) accentuated pulmonic valve closure sound (P_2)

153. Maldevelopment of the endocardial cushions may result in

(1) an atrial septal defect
(2) a ventricular septal defect
(3) deformity of the mitral valve
(4) deformity of the tricuspid valve

DIRECTIONS: Each group of questions below consists of lettered headings followed by a set of numbered items. For each numbered item select the **one** lettered heading with which it is **most** closely associated. Each lettered heading may be used **once, more than once, or not at all.**

Questions 154–157

For each syndrome listed below, select the major cardiovascular abnormality with which it is most likely to be associated.

(A) Atrial septal defect
(B) Ventricular septal defect
(C) Patent ductus arteriosus
(D) Supravalvular aortic stenosis
(E) Peripheral pulmonic stenosis

154. Ellis–van Creveld syndrome

155. Trisomy 18

156. Holt-Oram syndrome

157. Cri-du-chat syndrome

Questions 158–161

For each condition, select the most appropriate treatment.

(A) Packed red blood cells
(B) 5% albumin solution
(C) Whole blood
(D) 5% dextrose in water containing 40 mEq/L of sodium chloride and 20 mEq/L of potassium acetate
(E) None of the above

158. Severe anemia

159. Continuing massive bleeding in a patient in shock

160. Prevention of dehydration in a patient NPO prior to surgery

161. Circulatory collapse in a dehydrated infant

The Cardiovascular System
Answers

123.   The answer is C. *(Rudolph, ed 17. pp 1356–1357.)* An important noncardiac manifestation of digitalis toxicity in infants is vomiting. Affected infants also exhibit certain electrocardiographic changes, including sinus arrhythmia and a wandering pacemaker, paroxysmal tachycardia, and a heart rate of less than 100 beats per minute. The commonly used digitalis preparation in infants is digoxin. Digoxin blood levels of 2 ng per 100 ml or less are usually therapeutic in adults; in contrast, therapeutic digoxin blood levels in infants range from 1 to 5 ng per 100 ml, but the benefit of the higher levels in infants is doubtful.

124.   The answer is C. *(Behrman, ed 12. pp 298, 1167, 1502, 1638.)* Short stature, neck webbing, sexual infantilism, and a shieldlike chest with widely spaced nipples are signs of Turner's syndrome, which is usually associated with an XO karyotype. Aortic coarctation occurs most frequently in individuals who have this disorder. Down's syndrome most commonly is associated with endocardial cushion defects; Marfan's syndrome is associated with dilatation of the aorta and mitral and aortic regurgitation; and Ellis-van Creveld syndrome is associated with atrial septal defects.

125.   The answer is B. *(Behrman, ed 12. pp 1132–1134.)* Infants who have transposition of the great vessels classically present with cyanosis during the first few days after birth. Pulmonary vasculature is engorged. The cardiac contour in infants who have transposition has been described as an "egg on a string." The egg-shape is a result of general enlargement of the heart and the "string" is the narrow superior mediastinal shadow produced by the anteroposterior alignment of the aorta and main pulmonary artery.

126.   The answer is D. *(Keith, ed 3. p 4157. Roberts, p 390.)* The incidence of congenital heart disease in the population is 1 percent. The risk of congenital heart disease in a family with one child born with heart disease is 1 to 4 percent. If there are two children with congenital heart disease the risk escalates to 3 to 12 percent. Mothers with congenital heart disease have offspring with a 14-percent incidence of congenital heart disease. Children of mothers with congenital ventricular outflow obstruction have a 23-percent incidence of congenital heart defects.

127. The answer is A. *(Keith, ed 3. p 28.)* The harsh pansystolic murmur heard best in the third and fourth left intercostal spaces along the left sternal border and radiating to the apex is the classical murmur of a ventricular septal defect. An atrial septal defect would not cause a pansystolic murmur. Aortic and pulmonic regurgitation both cause diastolic murmurs, but neither has a rumbling quality. The aortic regurgitant flow may cause mitral vibrations heard at the apex. The quality is higher pitched and more likely blowing or harsh. Also these diastolic murmurs are heard in the pulmonic and aortic areas and may radiate down the sternal borders and, in the case of aortic stenosis, may be heard to the apex. A rumbling murmur that is very low pitched is usually generated across an atrioventricular valve. With both atrial and ventricular septal defects if the flow across the defect is large there may be a sufficiently large flow across the tricuspid valve (ASD) or mitral valve (VSD) to generate a diastolic rumbling murmur owing to relative atrioventricular valve stenosis. Because the baby has a pansystolic murmur and develops the rumbling apical murmur, he likely has progressively increasing flow from left to right across the ventricular septal defect.

128. The answer is A. *(Adams, ed 3. p 14.)* Although pulmonary arterioles are affected by pH and P_{CO_2} as well as by the presence of vasoactive substances, P_{O_2} is considered to be the major regulating influence of the pulmonary arteriolar resistance. The major smooth muscle relaxing effect of a high P_{O_2} causes pulmonary vascular resistance to fall.

129. The answer is C. *(Braunwald, ed 2. p 1053.)* All these conditions can be associated with prolonged fever and a limp caused by arthralgia, as well as exanthem, adenopathy, and pharyngitis. Conjunctivitis, however, is most likely in Kawasaki disease. The fissured lips, while common in Kawasaki disease, could occur after a long period of fever from any cause if the child became dehydrated. The predominance of neutrophils and high sedimentation rate are common to all. An increase in platelets, however, is found only in Kawasaki disease. Kawasaki disease presents a picture of prolonged fever, rash, epidermal peeling on the hands and feet, especially around the fingertips, ocular conjunctivitis, lymphadenopathy, fissured lips, oropharyngeal mucosal erythema, and arthralgia or arthritis. The diagnosis is still possible in the absence of one or two of these physical findings. Coronary artery aneurysms may develop.

130. The answer is A. *(Keith, ed 3. p 928–933.)* The findings of pallor, dyspnea, tachypnea, tachycardia, and cardiomegaly are common in congestive heart failure regardless of the cause. The lack of echocardiographic findings other than ventricular and left atrial dilation and poor ventricular function is inconsistent with both glycogen storage disease of the heart, in which there is muscle thickening, and pericarditis, since there is no pericardial effusion. It is also not consistent with an aberrant origin of the left coronary artery although the origin of the coronary arteries may be more easily missed. On electrocardiogram, the voltages of the ventricular complexes seen with aberrant origin of the left coronary artery are not diminished and a pattern of myocardial infarction may be seen. Voltages from the left ventricle are usually high in endocardial fibroelastosis, and both right and left ventricular forces are high in glycogen storage disease of the heart.

131. The answer is C. *(Braunwald, ed 2. p 1686.)* Hypoxic stimulation of the kidneys is thought to cause the release of erythropoietin that stimulates production of red blood cells in the bone marrow. A substrate manufactured in the liver is converted into erythropoietin, most likely in a reaction catalyzed by erythrogenin, an enzyme produced in the kidneys. Aside from inducing production of red blood cells, erythropoietin also causes the release of immature reticulocytes into the blood.

132. The answer is E. *(Adams, ed 3. p 733. Behrman, ed 12. pp 1171–1172.)* Congestive heart failure from any cause can result in mild cyanosis, even in the absence of a right-to-left shunt, and poor peripheral pulses when cardiac output is low. Congestive heart failure usually is associated with a rapid pulse rate (up to 200 beats per minute). A pulse rate greater than 200 beats per minute, however, should suggest the presence of a tachyarrhythmia.

133. The answer is A. *(Braunwald, ed 2. p 1626.)* Syncopal episodes in children are not common. Evaluation of children presenting with syncope should include electrocardiography, because arrhythmias can cause syncope. It is less likely that syncopy in a 3-year-old child would be caused by asymmetric septal hypertrophy; echocardiography is the procedure best able to evaluate this disorder.

134. The answer is D. *(Perloff, ed 2. pp 93–96, 119, 137.)* A loud systolic ejection murmur in the aortic area occurs with valvular, discrete subvalvular, and supravalvular aortic stenosis, but only supravalvular aortic stenosis is associated with these facial abnormalities. These patients are described as having elfin faces and very often suffer some degree of mental retardation. A bicuspid valve will more likely be associated with regurgitation and, therefore, a diastolic murmur. A brisk right brachial and weaker left brachial pulse are frequent findings in supravalvular aortic stenosis and are thought to be due to the jet of blood directed into the innominate artery by the supravalvular narrowing, causing the more prominent pulse on the right. For the same reason, the right arm blood pressure is about 10 to 15 mm higher than the left. With coarctation of the aorta, the left arm blood pressure and pulse may be less than in the right arm if the left subclavian artery is narrowed by the coarcted portion of the aorta. However, in aortic coarctation one would expect higher pressure in the right arm than in the leg.

135. The answer is A. *(Rudolph, ed 17. pp 1352–1358.)* The greatest cause of congestive heart failure in children is congenital heart disease. Congestive heart failure from congenital heart disease most often occurs in infants during their first weeks of life. Other etiologies of heart failure in young infants include primary myocardial disease, metabolic abnormalities, and paroxysmal atrial tachycardia; other causes, such as bacterial endocarditis and rheumatic heart disease, are rare in the first year of life.

136. The answer is C. *(Rudolph, ed 17. pp 1292–1294, 1313–1315.)* Children who have an atrial septal defect also may have right ventricular hypertrophy. A loud pulmonic component of the second sound occurs with development of pulmonary arterial hypertension. This may be reversible during childhood.

137. The answer is D. *(Rudolph, ed 17. pp 1329–1330.)* A quadruple rhythm associated with the murmur of tricuspid regurgitation and a middiastolic murmur at the lower left sternum suggests the diagnosis of Ebstein's anomaly (downward displacement of the tricuspid valve). The presence of P pulmonale (tall P waves in leads II and III) and right ventricular conduction defects confirms the diagnosis. Both tricuspid regurgitation with pulmonic stenosis and tetralogy of Fallot give electrocardiographic evidence of right ventricular enlargement. The Wolff-Parkinson-White syndrome, which frequently accompanies Ebstein's malformation, is not associated with murmurs or cyanosis as an isolated entity.

138. The answer is C. *(Keith, ed 3. pp 279, 286–288.)* The child described in the question, who has no cyanosis or murmur, no cardiac or pulmonary vascular abnormalities by chest x-ray, and no evidence of structural anomalies by echocardiogram, is unlikely to have an underlying gross anatomic defect. The electrocardiographic pattern in the figure shows the configuration of preexcitation, the pattern seen in the Wolff-Parkinson-White syndrome (WPW). These patients have an aberrant atrioventricular conduction pathway, which causes the early ventricular depolarization appearing on the electrocardiogram as a shortened PR interval. The initial slow ventricular depolarization wave is referred to as the delta wave. Seventy percent of patients with WPW have single or repeated episodes of paroxysmal supraventricular tachycardia, which can cause the symptoms described in the question. The preexcitation electrocardiographic pattern and WPW can occur in Ebstein's malformation, but this is unlikely in the absence of cyanosis and with a normal echocardiogram. Ventricular tachycardia is unlikely with WPW. If this were present, the symptoms would likely be more profound. Active play in a healthy 4-year-old child rarely causes symptoms such as those described in the question, but in children with WPW it can occasionally precipitate paroxysmal supraventricular tachycardia.

139. The answer is B. *(Behrman, ed 12. p 1175.)* During the first day of life, an infant's pulse rate can range from 70 to 180 beats per minute (average: 125); during the first week, the rate varies between 100 and 190 beats per minute (average: 140). A heart rate that persistently falls below 70 beats per minute almost invariably indicates congenital atrioventricular block, which is of the complete type in nearly all cases. Affected infants often present only with bradycardia; however, cyanosis, cardiomegaly, and heart failure can ensue, especially if the pulse rate falls below 50 beats per minute; these children would require cardiac pacing.

140. The answer is B. *(Behrman, ed 12. pp 564–572.)* Juvenile rheumatoid arthritis frequently causes spindle-shaped swelling of finger joints and may involve unusual joints such as the sternoclavicular joint. This disorder can be associated with spiking high fevers, which are not a feature of rheumatic fever, toxic synovitis, septic arthritis, or osteoarthritis. Although septic arthritis may affect any joint, it would not be likely to affect finger joints by causing spindle-shaped swellings; in this respect, septic arthritis resembles acute rheumatic fever. Toxic synovitis usually involves hip joints in boys, and osteoarthritis is not a disease of childhood.

141. The answer is B. *(Keith, ed 3. pp 487, 568.)* Transposition of the great vessels with an intact ventricular septum presents with early cyanosis, a normal-sized heart, normal or slightly increased pulmonary vascular markings, and an electrocardiogram showing right axis deviation and right ventricular hypertrophy. In tetralogy of Fallot, cyanosis is unlikely in the first few days of life. Tricuspid atresia, a cause of early cyanosis, causes diminished pulmonary arterial blood flow; the pulmonary fields on x-ray demonstrate a diminution of pulmonary vascularity. There is a left axis and left ventricular hypertrophy by electrocardiogram. Total anomalous pulmonary venous return below the diaphragm is associated with obstruction to pulmonary venous return and a classical radiographic finding of marked fluffy-appearing pulmonary venous congestion. In pulmonic atresia with intact ventricular septum, cyanosis appears early, the lung markings are normal to diminished, and the heart is large.

142. The answer is C. *(Ziai, ed 3. pp 254–255.)* Among the wide variety of cardiac defects associated with Down's syndrome, the most common are endocardial cushion defects and atrial septal defects. About half of all children with Down's syndrome are estimated to have congenital heart disease. Some cardiac lesions, such as tetralogy of Fallot and coarctation of the aorta, have been found to occur with less frequency in children who have Down's syndrome.

143. The answer is B (1,3). *(Braunwald, ed 2. p 948.)* Infants who are in congestive heart failure usually are hyperpneic, if they have hypoxemia and acidemia, or tachypneic, if they have volume overload of the pulmonary circuit. Grunting is associated primarily with pulmonary disease, and periodic breathing with disease or immaturity of the central nervous system.

144. The answer is E (all). *(Behrman, ed 12. pp 1139–1140.)* Aortic atresia, mitral atresia, and hypoplasia of the aortic arch, either individually or in combination along with hypoplasia of the left atrium and ventricle of varying degrees, constitute the hypoplastic left heart syndrome. Endocardial fibroelastosis is an associated defect, but it may also occur as an isolated finding without a small left ventricle.

145. The answer is A (1,2,3). *(Adams, ed 3. pp 268–269.)* Pulmonic stenosis usually is associated with a small-chambered right ventricle that, even following valvotomy, will not allow adequate blood flow into the pulmonary artery. Affected infants require maintenance of their aorticopulmonary shunts. Surgical aortico-pulmonary anastomosis, when possible, is the best treatment; infiltration of the ductus arteriosus with formalin has been used for patients who, for anatomical reasons, cannot undergo anastomosis. Prostaglandin (type E) infusion, a temporary emergency measure, can maintain ductal patency until surgery is performed.

146. The answer is A (1,2,3). *(Braunwald, ed 2. pp 824–825.)* The major factor in rapid fall of the pulmonary arterial resistance is pulmonary arterial vasodilation resulting from the increased P_{O_2} to which vessels are exposed. Inflation of the lungs allows the vessels to expand, which is the initial cause of reduction of the resistance. Ductus arteriosus closure, which is brought about by the increase in P_{O_2} plus the change in local prostaglandin, results in a fall in pulmonary arterial pressure. The enhanced volume caused by foramen ovale closure is noncontributory.

147. The answer is E (all). *(Behrman, ed 12. pp 396–397.)* Infants born to diabetic mothers commonly have hypoglycemia, hypocalcemia, and hyperinsulinemia; hyperbilirubinemia also is more common in these infants than in infants of nondiabetic mothers. Newborn infants who are severely hypoglycemic may develop profound congestive heart failure. Even without associated cardiac lesions, murmurs of tricuspid insufficiency may appear because of marked cardiac dilation and persistent fetal pulmonary circulation.

148. The answer is A (1,2,3). *(Behrman, ed 12. pp 592–593.)* Administration of salicylates and steroids can relieve the inflammatory manifestations of acute rheumatic fever. Steroids may be necessary to treat affected children who have carditis. Neither salicylates nor corticosteroids have an effect on chorea.

149. The answer is B (1,3). *(Keith, ed 3. pp 269, 279–280, 292, 700–701.)* In a child presenting with a seizure, cardiac causes, even though less likely than neurologic causes, must be considered. Ventricular arrhythmia may cause syncope resembling a seizure. Long Q-T syndrome, aortic stenosis, and primary hypertension can all cause ventricular fibrillation with stress. Atrial tachycardia may cause heart failure but does not cause syncope. If aortic stenosis were present, there would be a loud systolic ejection murmur with a thrill. The hearing deficit suggests the possibility of the Jervell and Lange-Nielsen syndrome, the recessive form of the long

Q-T syndrome, which is associated with a congenital hearing deficit. The mildly accentuated second sound is difficult to evaluate in a child with a thin chest wall, as is the recent onset of fatigue. These two findings, however, may be seen in pulmonary hypertension.

150. The answer is A (1,2,3). *(Rudolph, ed 17. pp 1285, 1323–1324, 1335, 1337.)* The continuous flow of blood through a truncus arteriosus into the pulmonary vessel gives rise to a continuous murmur. Similarly, the continuous blood flow through bronchial collateral vessels can cause a continuous murmur in children who have tetralogy of Fallot. In total anomalous pulmonary venous return, the flow through the pulmonary venous trunk carrying the blood from the pulmonary veins to the right heart may result in a continuous murmur. The murmur associated with patent ductus arteriosus is continuous and affected only to a minor degree by position or respiration, but patients are not cyanotic; in patent ductus arteriosus complicated by pulmonary hypertension, flow through the ductus is not continuous and, therefore, neither is the murmur.

151. The answer is E (all). *(Keith, ed 3. p 538.)* In all patients with tricuspid atresia there is need for a nonrestrictive communication across the atrial septum to allow the systemic venous return to the functioning ventricle. In addition these patients may require operative aorticopulmonary shunts to provide blood flow to the lungs. In the rare situations in which there is excessive blood flow into the pulmonary circuit, pulmonary banding may be necessary to reduce the excessive pulmonary flow.

152. The answer is B (1,3). *(Perloff, ed 3. pp 299–302.)* As in atrial septal defects, the increased flow across the pulmonic valve caused by the shunt causes a pulmonic flow murmur. The increased right ventricular volume results in a prominent right ventricular impulse (heave). The pulmonic second sound (P_2) is accentuated only in the presence of pulmonary hypertension. Wide and fixed splitting of the second heart sound, which classically occurs with atrial septal defects with significant flows, does not occur with the increased flow into the right atrium secondary to partial anomalous venous return with intact atrial septum.

153. The answer is E (all). *(Perloff, ed 3. pp 344–350.)* The embryonic endocardial cushions are responsible for the conjoining of the lower portion of the atrial septum and the upper portion of the ventricular septum, as well as the development of the anterior mitral leaflet and the septal leaflet of the tricuspid valve. Maldevelopment of the cushions can result, depending on degree, in a single or a combination of defects: atrial septal defect, ventricular septal defect, mitral or tricuspid regurgitation, or when severe, complete atrioventricular canal defect with communication of all four heart chambers.

154–157. The answers are: 154-A, 155-B, 156-A, 157-B. *(Braunwald, ed 2. p 943.)* The Ellis–van Creveld syndrome is an autosomal recessive trait. The common cardiac defects—often a secundum atrial septal defect—occur in 50 to 60 percent of affected individuals. This may be associated with some variant of hypoplastic left heart syndrome. The characteristic skeletal findings are short stature from birth, distal extremity shortening, and bilateral polydactyly. The last permits an in utero diagnosis.

The most common intracardiac defect in children with trisomy 18 is a ventricular septal defect. Patent ductus arteriosus is also commonly present. The cardiac defects are usually major and often result in heart failure, which is a significant factor in the early death of these children.

The Holt-Oram syndrome is one of the rare disorders in which a secundum atrial septal defect seems to be the result of a single dominant gene. Ventricular septal defect is the second most common cardiac anomaly. The most common hand/arm defect is a fingerlike appearance of one or both thumbs. First-degree relatives of patients with Holt-Oram syndrome have a 50-percent incidence of atrial septal defects, as opposed to a 3-percent occurrence in the sporadically occurring type of atrial septal defect.

Children with cri-du-chat syndrome have a chromosomal abnormality (5p −). The associated cardiac anomaly is a ventricular septal defect. There is microcephaly, an antimongoloid slant of the palpebral fissures, and severe mental retardation.

158–161. The answers are: 158-A, 159-C, 160-D, 161-B. *(Finberg, pp 141–145.)* With severe chronic anemia, plasma volume will already be expanded and it is, therefore, important to increase red-cell volume with a minimal increase in blood volume. This can be done by a partial exchange transfusion or by the slow infusion of packed red blood cells, allowing time for physiological mechanisms, involving the liver and kidney, to reduce plasma volume.

A patient in shock with continuing bleeding needs replacement of blood volume and this can be done best with whole blood or by administering both packed cells and plasma.

To prevent dehydration, a solution containing some glucose and small amounts of sodium, potassium, and basic anions will provide all that is needed for a few days. The other products would therefore be unnecessary and add the dangers associated with transfusion of blood and blood products.

With circulatory shock in a dehydrated infant, it is important to rapidly expand blood volume so that tissue perfusion improves and renal and cardiopulmonary systems can function to correct the disturbances that have been produced. Of the solutions given, the 5% albumin solution would be best, but if the patient was also anemic, then whole blood or packed cells could also be used if it could be made available quickly enough. Solution D would not be appropriate, since it is too low in sodium to expand extracellular volume adequately. A solution with a higher sodium concentration in the range of 90 to 150 mEq/L, however, could be used.

The Respiratory System

DIRECTIONS: Each question below contains five suggested responses. Select the **one best** response to each question.

162. A previously well 1-year-old infant has had a runny nose and had been sneezing and coughing for 2 days. Two other members of the family had similar symptoms. Four hours ago his cough became much worse. On physical examination he is in moderate respiratory distress with nasal flaring, hyperexpansion of the chest, and easily audible wheezing without rales. The most likely diagnosis is

— (A) bronchiolitis
  (B) viral croup
  (C) asthma
  (D) epiglottitis
  (E) diphtheria

163. The most likely etiologic agent responsible for the infant's condition in the previous question is

  (A) *Staphylococcus aureus*
  (B) *Haemophilus influenzae*
  (C) *Corynebacterium diphtheriae*
— (D) respiratory syncytial virus
  (E) ECHO virus

164. A 13-year-old girl with a history of 2 days of cough and fever has the chest x-ray shown below. The most appropriate treatment is

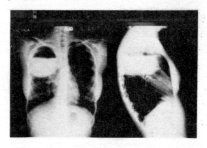

  (A) *N*-acetylcysteine
— (B) penicillin 100,000 U/kg per day
      for 1 month
  (C) lobectomy
  (D) postural drainage
  (E) thoracentesis and chest tube

66

165. A small, thin 12-year-old boy with a chronic cough has the chest x-ray below. The most likely x-ray diagnosis is

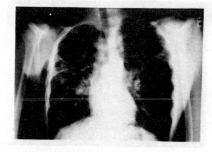

(A) asthma
(B) bronchiolitis
(C) croup
— (D) bronchiectasis
(E) pulmonary hemosiderosis

166. In the patient in the previous question, underlying diseases that should be considered in the differential diagnosis are listed below. The one that is most likely is

(A) foreign body aspiration
— (B) cystic fibrosis
(C) immotile cilia syndrome
(D) measles
(E) immunodeficiency syndrome

167. If one child in a family has cystic fibrosis, and neither parent has the disease, the chance of a subsequent child having cystic fibrosis is

(A) 5 percent
(B) 15 percent
(C) 25 percent
(D) 50 percent
(E) 100 percent

168. The etiology of the sudden infant death syndrome is

(A) prolonged apnea
(B) cardiac irregularity
(C) immaturity of the brainstem
(D) excess endorphins
— (E) unknown

169. The average death rate attributed to SIDS per 100,000 live births in the United States is

(A) 0.2
(B) 2
(C) 20
— (D) 200
(E) 2,000

170. Clinical trials have shown that SIDS may be prevented by

(A) apnea monitoring
(B) cardiac monitoring
(C) polysomnography
(D) theophylline administration
— (E) none of the above

171. An otherwise well 3-year-old girl with a strongly positive tuberculin test should be treated with

—(A) isoniazid for 1 year
(B) isoniazid for 1 year and streptomycin for 1 month
(C) isoniazid for 1 year, streptomycin for 1 month, and ethambutol for 6 months
(D) ethambutol for 6 months and rifampin for 6 months
(E) pyridoxine for 1 year

172. The patient in the previous question comes back 2 months later with fever for the past week, irritability, and vomiting. The mother tells you she gave the child isoniazid for only 1 week and then stopped it. Physical examination is unrevealing. The next step should be to

(A) administer thorazine
(B) do lumbar puncture
(C) repeat tuberculin test
(D) get repeat chest x-ray
(E) get psychiatric consultation for the family

173. A patient with staphylococcal pneumonia suddenly develops increasing respiratory distress. The possible diagnosis requiring the most urgent action is

(A) pneumatocele formation
(B) tension pneumothorax
(C) progression of the pneumonia
(D) severe anxiety
(E) pleural effusion

174. Following a chest x-ray that showed a right-sided tension pneumothorax, the patient in the previous question has developed even worse respiratory distress and is now deeply cyanotic in 80% oxygen. The best course would be to

(A) increase oxygen to 90%
(B) request surgical consultation for chest tube placement
(C) give intravenous bicarbonate
(D) follow blood gases
(E) use needle and syringe to do emergency decompression

175. A 3-year-old boy has a young puppy and a history of pica. He has had the recent onset of wheezing, hepatomegaly, and marked eosinophilia (80 percent eosinophils). The test most likely to produce a specific diagnosis is

(A) tuberculin skin test
(B) histoplasmin test
(C) ELISA for *Toxocara*
(D) silver stain of gastric aspirate
(E) stool examination for ova and parasites

176. You receive a telephone call from the reliable mother of a 4-year-old child with sickle cell anemia. She tells you that the child is breathing fast, coughing, and has a temperature of 103°F. The most conservative, prudent approach is to

(A) prescribe aspirin and ask her to call back if the fever does not respond
(B) make an office appointment for the next available opening
(C) make an office appointment for the next day
(D) refer the child to the laboratory for an immediate hematocrit, white blood cell count, and differential
(E) admit the child to the hospital as an emergency

177. You see the patient of the previous question in the hospital one-half hour later and you find her as the mother described. Although the patient is in respiratory distress, the lack of cyanosis indicates

(A) that there is not significant hypoxia
(B) that the patient has pulmonary thrombi rather than pneumonia
(C) very little since it is not a useful indication of hypoxia in a patient with anemia
(D) shift of the oxyhemoglobin curve to the right owing to increased levels of DPG
(E) an adequate hemoglobin level for the given activity level

178. The laboratory workup of the patient of the previous question reveals the following: hemoglobin 6 g/100 ml; hematocrit 19; white blood cell count 30,000/mm^3; arterial blood while breathing room air—pH 7.1, P_{O_2} 35 mm Hg; P_{CO_2} 28 mm Hg. This indicates

(A) acidemia, metabolic acidosis, respiratory alkalosis, hypoxia
(B) alkalemia, respiratory acidosis, metabolic alkalosis, hypoxia
(C) acidosis with compensatory hypoventilation
(D) long-term metabolic compensation for respiratory alkalosis
(E) primary respiratory alkalosis

179. While waiting for further studies of the patient of the previous question, it is appropriate to

(A) give sedation
(B) give bicarbonate by IV push
(C) give urea
(D) administer 100% oxygen
(E) administer 40% oxygen with 5% carbon dioxide

180. During the past 8 months, a 15-year-old boy has had seven episodes typified by sudden onset of severe respiratory distress with fever and malaise. Chest x-rays at the times of the episodes show transient patchy infiltrates. Etiologic factors to be considered include

(A) moist hay
(B) cane sugar fiber
(C) pigeon droppings
(D) home humidifiers
(E) all of the above

181. A 4-year-old boy with asthma who is on an IV aminophylline drip is finally sleeping after having been in respiratory distress all day. On auscultation of the chest you hear only slight wheezing. Vital signs are normal except for mild tachypnea. You should now

(A) order vital signs every one-half hour
(B) repeat the chest x-ray
(C) get an allergy consultation
(D) get an arterial blood gas
(E) continue theophylline and get a serum level

DIRECTIONS: Each question below contains four suggested responses of which **one or more** is correct. Select

A	if	**1, 2, and 3**	are correct
B	if	**1 and 3**	are correct
C	if	**2 and 4**	are correct
D	if	**4**	is correct
E	if	**1, 2, 3, and 4**	are correct

182. Cystic fibrosis involves which of the following organs?

(1) Lungs
(2) Liver
(3) Pancreas
(4) Intestines

183. Reasonable explanations for an elevated chloride concentration (136 mEq/L) in the sweat of a 3-year-old boy with recurrent pneumonias include that

(1) he has cystic fibrosis
(2) he has ectodermal dysplasia
(3) the skin was not washed properly to remove residual salt before the collection of sweat was begun
(4) this is the upper limit of normal

184. You are wakened in the night by your 2-year-old who has developed noisy breathing on inspiration, marked retractions of the chest wall, flaring of the nostrils, and a barking cough. He has previously been well except for a mild URI that day. Diagnoses that should be seriously considered are

(1) asthma
(2) epiglottitis
(3) bronchiolitis
(4) viral croup

185. In the situation described in the previous question, appropriate actions would be to

(1) look at the epiglottis with a flashlight using the handle of a spoon in the absence of appropriate equipment
(2) give syrup of ipecac and place the child in the bathroom with the shower turned on
(3) provide sedation to relieve the anxiety and encourage sleep
(4) call the child's physician and meet her at the nearest emergency room capable of dealing with this problem

186. Infections with *Mycoplasma pneumonia* can produce which of the following?

(1) Lobar pneumonia
(2) Bronchopneumonia
(3) Tracheobronchitis
(4) Otitis media

187. *Chlamydia trachomatis* infections of infants produce

(1) conjunctivitis
(2) urethritis
(3) pneumonia
(4) encephalitis

188. Appropriate treatment of chlamydial pneumonia in a 6-week-old infant includes

(1) penicillin
(2) tetracycline
(3) amphotericin B
(4) erythromycin

189. During routine screening for tuberculosis a 3-year-old girl has been found to have a strongly positive tuberculin test. This indicates

(1) exposure to an adult with tuberculosis
(2) need for testing of family members
(3) infection with tuberculosis
(4) need for isolation of the child

190. Typical findings in the cerebrospinal fluid of a patient with tuberculous meningitis include

(1) 90 white blood cells per mm³, 60 percent lymphocytes
(2) glucose 10 mg per 100 ml
(3) protein 80 mg per 100 ml
(4) cloudiness

191. Patients who are on isoniazid should be followed to look for evidence of development of adverse reactions. These present as

(1) jaundice
(2) rash
(3) fever
(4) peripheral neuritis

192. Characteristics of the chest x-ray in staphylococcal pneumonia include

(1) pneumatoceles
(2) pleural effusion
(3) rapid progression
(4) pneumothorax

193. You are considering the possibility that your patient may need emergency endotracheal intubation. Before being used the laryngoscope should be checked for

(1) a loose bulb
(2) dead batteries
(3) proper-sized blades
(4) sterility

194. One can approximate the size of the endotracheal tube needed for a patient since the diameter of the glottis is close to the diameter of the patient's

(1) little finger
(2) external ear canal
(3) external nares
(4) fully dilated pupil

195. After endotracheal intubation, it is appropriate to check the position of the tube by

(1) chest x-ray
(2) auscultation for symmetrical breath sounds
(3) fiberoptic endoscopy
(4) instillation of saline while listening for bubbling sounds

196. Systemic infection with *Histoplasma capsulatum* produces a wide spectrum of illness that can be mistaken for

(1) tuberculosis
(2) leukemia
(3) ulcerative colitis
(4) bacterial endocarditis

197. Recommendations for treatment of histoplasmosis include

(1) penicillin
(2) amphotericin B
(3) streptomycin
(4) sulfonamides

198. A 10-year-old boy with progressive bronchopneumonia, high fever and chills, and no bacteria on gram stain of sputum, and who continues to worsen despite therapy with ampicillin has characteristics of disease caused by

(1) *Mycoplasma pneumoniae*
(2) influenza virus
(3) *Legionella pneumophila*
(4) chlamydia

DIRECTIONS: Each group of questions below consists of lettered headings followed by a set of numbered items. For each numbered item select the **one** lettered heading with which it is **most** closely associated. Each lettered heading may be used **once, more than once, or not at all.**

Questions 199–202

Match each management procedure below with the appropriate arterial blood gas results of patients spontaneously breathing room air.

	pH	P_{CO_2} (mm Hg)	P_{O_2} (mm Hg)	Base Excess (mEq/L)
(A)	7.20	28	95	−16
(B)	7.20	70	41	−2
(C)	7.64	18	94	−1
(D)	7.34	32	39	−8
(E)	None of the above			

C 199. Have patient rebreathe in a paper bag

D 200. Administer FIO_2 0.4

A 201. Expand blood volume to normal

B 202. Perform thoracentesis to remove air under pressure

Questions 203–206

Match each management procedure below with the appropriate arterial blood gas results of patients spontaneously breathing room air.

	pH	P_{CO_2} (mm Hg)	P_{O_2} (mm Hg)	Base Excess (mEq/L)
(A)	6.92	101	19	−15
(B)	7.36	60	50	+7
(C)	7.50	46	76	+11
(D)	7.41	60	90	+10
(E)	None of the above			

A 203. Place the patient on a ventilator with an FIO_2 of 1.0

C 204. Discontinue diuretics, discontinue base and increase KCl in IV fluids

B 205. Perform tonsillectomy

D 206. Repeat the test because of obvious laboratory error

DIRECTIONS: The group of questions below consists of four lettered headings followed by a set of numbered items. For each numbered item select

A	if the item is associated with	(A) **only**
B	if the item is associated with	(B) **only**
C	if the item is associated with	**both** (A) and (B)
D	if the item is associated with	**neither** (A) nor (B)

Each lettered heading may be used **once, more than once, or not at all.**

Questions 207–210

(A) Retropharyngeal abscess
(B) Retrotonsillar abscess
(C) Both
(D Neither

C 207. Complication of acute pharyngitis

B 208. Likely in children over 4 years old

C 209. Cause of pharyngeal bulge

C 210. Surgical treatment required

The Respiratory System
Answers

162. The answer is A. *(Behrman, ed 12. pp 1044-1045.)* Of the choices given, bronchiolitis is the most likely, although asthma, pertussis, and bronchopneumonia can present similarly. The family history of upper respiratory infections, the previous upper respiratory illness in the patient, and signs of intrathoracic airway obstruction make the diagnosis of bronchiolitis more likely. Since there are no signs of extrathoracic airway obstruction, viral croup, epiglottitis, and diphtheria are not reasonable choices.

163. The answer is D. *(Behrman, ed 12. p 1044.)* The most likely cause of the illness is respiratory syncytial virus infection, which causes outbreaks of bronchiolitis of varying severity, usually in the winter and spring. Other viruses such as parainfluenza and the adenoviruses have also been implicated in producing bronchiolitis. Treatment is usually supportive in this usually self-limited condition.

164. The answer is B. *(Behrman, ed 12. p 1073.)* The x-ray reveals a lung abscess involving the right upper lobe characterized by the round density, the air-fluid level, and the opaque rim. Lung abscesses are usually caused by anaerobic bacteria such as bacteroides, fusobacteria, and anaerobic streptococci, and on occasion by *Staphylococcus aureus* and *Klebsiella*. The organisms are often sensitive to penicillin. Lung abscesses frequently respond surprisingly well to treatment with antibiotics alone.

165. The answer is D. *(Behrman, ed 12. pp 1071-1073, 1086-1099.)* The x-ray shows rounded and linear densities in both lungs, worse on the right, which are typical of cylindrical and saccular bronchiectasis. Bronchiectasis is usually secondary to chronic bacterial infection of the bronchi with damage to the bronchial walls with dilatation and collection of suppurative material. Bronchiectasis is rarely congenital.

166. The answer is B. *(Behrman, ed 12. pp 1071–1073.)* Before effective immunization practices became widespread and before the advent of effective antibiotic treatment of infections, bronchiectasis was a relatively common condition and frequently complicated measles, pertussis, and bacterial pneumonia. It is now most commonly seen in patients with cystic fibrosis, but the other diagnoses listed are also possible. Other etiologies include dysautonomia, gastroesophageal reflux, tuberculosis, sarcoidosis, and neoplasms.

167. The answer is C. *(Behrman, ed 12. p. 1086.)* Cystic fibrosis appears to be inherited as an autosomal recessive trait, so that the risk to subsequent offspring of heterozygotic parents is that 1 in 4 will have the disease. One half will be carriers and 1 in 4 will not carry the gene. Four to five percent of whites carry the gene but the disease incidence varies from 1:682 in Afrikaners to 1:90,000 in Asians in Hawaii. In the United States it occurs in 1:2,000 whites and 1:17,000 blacks.

168. The answer is E. *(Rudolph, ed 17. pp 768–772.)* There have been many theories as to the etiology of the sudden infant death syndrome (SIDS), but none have been substantiated. A large number of studies have been done and are in progress looking at those possibilities listed in the question, as well as others involving deficiencies in thiamine, vitamins D and E, and selenium, *Clostridium botulinum* infection, and defective gluconeogenesis, so we are continually learning more about SIDS. It is important to remember that just because we can give something a name and generate multiple hypotheses does not mean we know very much about it.

169. The answer is D. *(Rudolph, ed 17. pp 768–773.)* The death rate for SIDS is usually cited as 2 per 1,000 in the United States, but this varies somewhat from place to place and among social and racial groups. It is more common among the poor, in blacks, in premature infants, in the winter, and at night. It predominantly affects infants between 1 and 5 months of age and peaks at around 3 months.

170. The answer is E. *(Rudolph, ed 17. pp 768–773.)* None of the measures developed to prevent SIDS has yet to be demonstrated by clinical trials to be effective. Nevertheless, electronic apnea and cardiac monitoring with appropriate alarm settings are rational approaches to infants who may be at high risk for SIDS, such as those who have had a sibling with SIDS or a "near miss" for SIDS. In these situations the parents' high anxiety level would often have them performing 24-hour respiratory and cardiac monitoring, anyway, and the electronic devices make it easier for them.

171. The answer is A. *(Ziai, ed 3. p. 494.)* It may be assumed that young children with a strongly positive tuberculin test have active disease and require, at least, treatment with isoniazid for 1 year. The reason for the treatment is not to treat the current illness, which usually resolves spontaneously, but to prevent later complications. In such patients with minimal disease isoniazid alone is adequate.

172. The answer is B. *(Ziai, ed 3. pp 488–489.)* Families do not always follow their physician's advice, which points out the need for effective transmission of information and for careful followup. Since the nonspecific symptoms in the question may be early signs of tuberculous meningitis, they mandate prompt performance of lumbar puncture in search of signs of meningitis. If there are indications of elevated intracranial pressure, a CAT scan, with contrast, of the head may be done first. In tuberculous meningitis the exudate at the base of the brain enhances with the contrast medium.

173. The answer is B. *(Ziai, ed 3. pp 222–224.)* Tension pneumothorax, a well-recognized complication of staphylococcal pneumonia, can be quickly lethal and is easily treated. This makes a high index of suspicion and prompt diagnosis mandatory. The other complications can occur also but do not require as prompt a response.

174. The answer is E. *(Rudolph, ed 17. pp 1409–1410.)* Cyanosis while breathing high concentrations of oxygen indicates severe respiratory compromise with right to left shunting of blood, and death is imminent. No time remains to do more diagnostic procedures or to get help. Immediate action to relieve the tension is mandatory. This can easily be done by inserting a needle or catheter into the second or third intercostal spaces in the midclavicular line, with the patient supine. A three-way stopcock on the syringe is an added refinement.

175. The answer is C. *(Kendig, ed 4. pp 835–837.)* The presentation described is characteristic of visceral larva migrans from infestation with the common parasite of dogs *Toxocara canis*. Dirt-eating children ingest the infectious ova. The larvae penetrate the intestine and migrate to visceral sites, such as the liver, lung, and brain, but do not return to the intestine, so the stools do not contain the ova or parasites. There has recently been developed a specific enzyme-linked immunosorbent assay (ELISA) for *Toxocara*.

176. The answer is E. *(Kendig, ed 4. pp 884–896.)* Fever, cough, and tachypnea in a patient with sickle cell anemia may be manifestations of pneumonia, pulmonary thromboemboli, or sepsis. Aside from being relatively common in patients with sickle cell anemia these diseases may be rapidly progressive and quickly fatal. It is therefore important for the patient to be evaluated and treated on an emergency basis. The treatment requires hospitalization since it will almost certainly include systemic antibiotics, intravenous fluids, oxygen, and perhaps blood transfusion.

177. The answer is C. *(Finberg, p 39.)* In order to see cyanosis there must be about 5 g of unoxygenated hemoglobin in the skin capillaries. In anemia this may not be possible since the total hemoglobin level may be beneath that. In addition, dark skin pigmentation and poor lighting contribute to making cyanosis an unreliable negative sign. With anemia and pulmonary disease one should assume the patient has impaired oxygenation.

178. The answer is A. *(Finberg, pp 35–55.)* The low pH in the arterial blood can be called acidemia. In this context it is likely that the hydrogen ions come from lactic acid produced by anaerobic metabolism in tissues with inadequate oxygen delivery. Inadequate oxygenation is caused by the low P_{o_2}, the low oxygen-carrying capacity of the blood (Hb 6 g per 100 ml), and by circulatory inadequacy owing to the sickling itself and to the vascular disease it produces. The low P_{co_2} reflects the hyperventilation, which is secondary to the hypoxia, to the respiratory difficulty, and to the anemia, and is also respiratory compensation for the metabolic acidosis.

179. The answer is D. *(Finberg, p 38.)* Administration of 100% oxygen will rapidly raise alveolar oxygen concentration and in the absence of substantial right to left shunting of blood will fully saturate the arterial hemoglobin. It will also dissolve 0.003 ml of oxygen per mm Hg of oxygen partial pressure in each deciliter of blood. This will serve to decrease the tissue hypoxia, and increase the mixed venous oxygen concentration, which may decrease the amount of sickling. Giving a patient like this 100% oxygen to breathe is the physiological equivalent in oxygen transportation capacity to a transfusion of 10 ml/kg of whole blood. This is only useful as a temporary measure since oxygen toxicity will start to develop after several hours. The other choices are all undesirable.

180. The answer is E. *(Kendig, ed 4. pp 544–564. Scarpelli, pp 536–537.)* The clinical findings are those of what has been termed hypersensitivity pneumonitis, extrinsic allergic alveolitis, or hypersensitivity alveolitis, but the last two names are misleading since the disease involves not only the alveoli, but the small airways and the interstitium of the lung as well. The illness is secondary to the inhalation of tiny particles of a variety of antigens of biological origin that reach the distal parts of the lungs. The best treatment is avoidance of the agent, but corticosteroids may be effective.

181. The answer is D. *(Finberg, pp 206–211.)* A decrease in wheezing in a patient with asthma is not always a sign of improvement, but may occur as hypoventilation develops. The rising levels of carbon dioxide initially produce excitement and increased respiratory effort, but then depression of brain activity, which may look like normal sleep with little apparent respiratory effort, develops as P_{co_2} continues to rise. This lack of both air flow and respiratory effort may eliminate wheezing. This situation is very deceptive and obviously very dangerous. An arterial blood gas would indicate the hypoventilation, and resuscitative measures could then follow.

182. The answer is E (all). *(Finberg, pp 212–218.)* Exocrine secretions are abnormal in cystic fibrosis and this leads to damage, directly or indirectly, to a variety of otherwise seemingly disparate parts of the body. The most devastating impact is on the lungs: chronic lung disease often leads to ventilatory failure. Digestive disturbances and malabsorption lead to nutritional deficiencies. Pancreatic fibrosis and cirrhosis of the liver may develop later.

183. The answer is A (1, 2, 3). *(Finberg, pp 212–216.)* Unlike many other tests there is almost no overlap in sweat chloride values between patients with cystic fibrosis and normal controls. A sweat chloride of 136 mEq/L is clearly above normal, which ranges to 50 mEq/L. The other explanations given are reasonable and the test should be repeated before a final diagnosis is made.

184. The answer is C (2, 4). *(Behrman, ed 12. pp 1034–1037.)* The signs of illness described are those involving the airway above the point at which the trachea enters the neck and leaves the thorax. Intrathoracic airway diseases, such as asthma or bronchiolitis, produce breathing difficulty on expiration with expiratory wheezing, prolonged expiration, and signs of air trapping owing to the increased narrowing during expiration as the airways are exposed to the same intrathoracic pressure changes as the alveoli. The extrathoracic airway, to the contrary, tends to collapse on inspiration, producing the characteristic findings that this patient has.

185. The answer is D (4). *(Behrman, ed 12. pp 1034–1035.)* Since epiglottitis is a reasonable possibility, the only appropriate course of action is to get the child to a place where the equipment and personnel are available to establish an emergency airway, if necessary, by endotracheal intubation, tracheostomy, cricothyroid stab, or by use of a large bore needle or catheter. Attempts to look at the throat of such a patient in an area not so staffed and equipped is dangerous since this may precipitate immediate, total airway obstruction. The use of sedation is an error in a patient with respiratory distress since it may worsen hypoventilation and would be totally inappropriate here. Administration of syrup of ipicac would just waste time.

186. The answer is E (all). *(Kendig, ed 4. pp 340–345.)* Infections with *Mycoplasma pneumoniae* are common in older children and young adults. Although the infection typically produces lower lobe bronchopneumonia, its effects are characteristically nonspecific and it can produce lobar pneumonia as well. It also can produce upper respiratory infection, pharyngitis, otitis media and externa, bronchiolitis, hemolytic anemia, and Guillain-Barré syndrome.

187. The answer is B (1, 3). *(Kendig, ed 4. p 767.)* Chlamydiae, sexually transmitted among adults, are spread to infants during birth from genitally infected mothers. The sites of infection in infants are the lungs and the conjunctivae where chlamydiae cause afebrile pneumonia and inclusion conjunctivitis in infants between 2 to 12 weeks of age. Diagnosis is confirmed by culture of nasopharyngeal secretions and by antibody titers.

188. The answer is D (4). *(Kendig, ed 4. p 770.)* Erythromycin is recommended for the treatment of chlamydial pneumonia. Sulfisoxazole may also be used. In addition, for ill infants, suctioning, postural drainage, oxygen, IV fluids, and apnea monitoring may also be indicated.

189. The answer is A (1, 2, 3). *(Ziai, ed 3. pp 484–486.)* The finding of a positive tuberculin test in a child indicates that there has been exposure to an adult with an infectious form of tuberculosis. This finding should set off a search for the source by taking a careful family, social, and environmental history, and doing tuberculin testing and chest x-rays of the family and close contacts. Primary tuberculosis in children is not considered a contagious illness and does not require isolation.

190. The answer is A (1,2,3). *(Ziai, ed 3. p 488.)* The spinal fluid tends to be clear in tuberculous meningitis with the white blood cell count ranging from 10 to 350 per mm^3, the majority being lymphocytes on differential examination. Glucose levels may be only slightly lower than normal early on in the disease and may get extremely low as the disease progresses. Protein levels follow the opposite course, being slightly elevated early on and then going higher, particularly with advanced disease and even more so with blockage to the flow of cerebrospinal fluid.

191. The answer is E (all). *(Goodman, ed 7. pp 1201–1202.)* Although isoniazid has a large number of adverse effects, most patients have an uneventful course. The incidence of hepatic disease is a function of age, being very rare in infants and children and occurring in 0.3 percent of those 20 to 34 years old and in 2.3 percent of those over 50. Elevation of transaminases is more common than symptomatic liver disease and an elevation five times normal is an indication to stop isoniazid. Pyridoxine is used to prevent peripheral neuritis in adults and older adolescents who are taking isoniazid, but is not necessary in infants and children. Hypersensitivity reactions such as skin eruptions and fever may also develop with use of isoniazid.

192. The answer is E (all). *(Ziai, ed 3. pp 222–223.)* Staphylococcal pneumonia requires specific therapy and will not generally respond well to the usual therapy for the other varieties of bacterial pneumonia; therefore, it is important to make this diagnosis as early as possible. The chest x-ray is frequently helpful in that the listed characteristics may be seen. They can be seen with other pneumonias as well, but finding them should alert one to the possibility of staphylococcal pneumonia and use of an antistaphylococcal penicillin should be strongly considered.

193. The answer is A (1,2,3). *(Levin, ed 2. pp 536–537.)* The tendency toward entropy is great for laryngoscopes; they often require mending. In addition to checking the laryngoscope for function prior to use, it is important to have back-up equipment. Sterility is not necessary, though cleanliness is desirable.

194. The answer is B (1,3). *(Levin, ed 2. p 536. Welch, ed 4. p 136.)* Before endotracheal intubation is attempted a variety of endotracheal tube sizes should be available so that the appropriately sized tube can be selected. The external diameter of the tube to be used can be approximated by comparing it with the size of the patient's external nares or little finger. The next sizes up and down should be readily available. Too small a tube will make ventilation and suctioning difficult and too large a tube will be placed with difficulty and will traumatize the larynx and trachea.

195. The answer is A (1,2,3). *(Kendig, ed 4. p 159.)* If endotracheal tube placement is too high, the tube may easily become misplaced into the esophagus. If it is down too far, it may enter the right main stem bronchus, prevent ventilation of the left lung, and allow excess volume to enter the right lung. This may lead to atelectasis and pneumothorax. Too low a position makes suctioning of the left lung difficult. Newer, narrower, fiberoptic endoscopes may replace chest x-rays for determining tube position.

196. The answer is E (all). *(Kendig, ed 4. pp 728–729.)* Histoplasmosis is a world-wide disease and is the most common systemic fungus infection. It is regionally distributed in the United States with the highest prevalence in Ohio, Indiana, Kentucky, Tennessee, Arkansas, Missouri, and the southern part of Illinois. In these areas and when caring for patients who have traveled from these areas, histoplasmosis should enter the differential diagnosis of those diseases listed in the question. It may mimic virtually all aspects of tuberculosis except for the negative tuberculin and positive histoplasmin skin tests.

197. The answer is C (2,4). *(Kendig, ed 4. pp 730, 754–755.)* Penicillin and streptomycin increase the growth of *Histoplasma capsulatum* in vitro and are therefore probably contraindicated. Amphotericin B and sulfonamides are recommended for treatment. Because amphotericin B is the most toxic antimicrobial agent in use (locally known as "amphoterrible"), it should be reserved for progressively invasive disease. It causes inflammation of veins, gastrointestinal disturbance, muscle and joint pain, hypertension, cardiac arrhythmias including cardiac arrest, anaphylaxis, anemia, and hypokalemia; it is hepatotoxic and nephrotoxic.

198. The answer is A (1,2,3). *(Kendig, ed 4. pp 810–821.)* Chlamydial pneumonia is afebrile. All the others are compatible with the clinical picture. Although Legionnaires' disease is rare in the pediatric age group, it does occur on occasion and has a high mortality when untreated. Diagnostic workup for these illnesses and treatment with erythromycin should be considered. Erythromycin is indicated in mycoplasma infections as well as those from legionella (and chlamydia).

199–202. The answers are: 199-C, 200-D, 201-A, 202-B. *(Finberg, pp 35–55, 91–107. Kravath, Pediatrics 59:865, 1977.)* The laboratory results of row C indicate a striking respiratory alkalosis. This could be secondary to voluntary hyperventilation or inappropriate respirator settings for a patient on a ventilator and is also typical of acute hyperventilation syndrome secondary to anxiety. Such a patient may complain of dyspnea, chest pain, tingling, and dizziness and may even have generalized convulsions secondary to low ionized calcium levels. Rebreathing into a paper bag may be both therapeutic and diagnostic.

The blood gases of row D are the only ones given that are relatively normal except for a low oxygen partial pressure. The mild respiratory alkalosis and metabolic acidosis may be a consequence of the hypoxia. These results could be obtained in a patient with moderately severe pneumonia, bronchiolitis, or asthma secondary to ventilation/perfusion inequality with some areas of the lung being underventilated with respect to perfusion. This cause of hypoxia may be easily corrected by giving the patient relatively small increases in oxygen concentration to breathe. These results would also be typical of findings in patients with right to left shunting of blood as in tetralogy of Fallot, in which case giving oxygen would not help (but cardiac surgery was not one of the options given to you in this question).

The results in row A show fairly severe metabolic acidosis with respiratory compensation and without hypoxia. These would be typical for someone in early shock and would most commonly be seen in children and in patients with diarrhea. The proper sequence of treatment of this type of acidosis, as proposed by Dr. William Segar, is (1) hydration, (2) hydration, and (3) hydration.

The blood gases of row B demonstrate an uncompensated respiratory acidosis with hypoxia but with no metabolic acidosis. This is compatible with acute hypoventilation, which could be produced by a tension pneumothorax, for example. This could easily be treated by placing a needle or catheter in the pleural space and evacuating the air.

203–206. The answers are: 203-A, 204-C, 205-B, 206-D. *(Finberg, pp 35–55, 91–107. Kravath, Pediatrics 59:865, 1977.)* The data on row A indicate severe acidemia and severe hypoxia with a marked respiratory acidosis and metabolic acidosis. These are manifestations of severe ventilatory failure, probably accompanied by circulatory failure or cardiac arrest. This mandates the most aggressive therapy, including assisted ventilation with administration of high oxygen levels. Other measures to restore circulation and improve the acidemia are also indicated.

The results of row C show metabolic alkalosis. The high P_{co_2} and low P_{o_2} result from compensatory hypoventilation. This can all be secondary to excessive body potassium losses from diuretics.

The results in row B indicate moderate metabolic alkalosis with almost complete compensation, indicating chronic upper airway obstruction. A common cause of chronic hypoventilation in children is hypertrophied tonsils and adenoids, which is an indication for tonsillectomy or adenoidectomy (or both).

The blood gases of row D are impossible in a patient breathing room air. The P_{co_2} cannot go up without the P_{o_2} dropping roughly proportionately. An increase in P_{co_2} of 20 mm Hg from 40 to 60 mm Hg should therefore produce a fall in P_{o_2} from 90 to 70 mm Hg. The test should be repeated after the blood gas equipment has been checked and recalibrated.

207–210. The answers are: 207-C, 208-B, 209-C, 210-C. *(Behrman, ed 12. pp 1017–1018.)* Both retropharyngeal and retrotonsillar abscesses can cause acute airway obstruction and erosion into vital structures and, therefore, require prompt diagnosis and treatment. Retropharyngeal abscess is more common in younger children (under 4 years of age) and retrotonsillar abscess is more common in older children. They usually represent complications of acute bacterial pharyngitis. *Staphylococcus aureus* and beta-hemolytic streptococci are the usual pathogens. When the abscess is fluctuant, incision and drainage under general anethesia is indicated in order to avoid aspiration of pus and airway compromise. To prevent recurrences, retrotonsillar or peritonsillar abscess is an indication for elective tonsillectomy when the infection has cleared.

Diagnosis can be made by the history of a prior pharyngitis with sudden worsening of symptoms, increasing fever, and the development of respiratory distress and difficulty in swallowing. Physical examination will reveal the typical bulging of the pharynx and fluctuance may be apparent on palpation.

The Gastrointestinal Tract

DIRECTIONS: Each question below contains five suggested responses. Select the **one best** response to each question.

211. All the following factors are associated with an increased risk of neurologic damage in a jaundiced newborn EXCEPT

(A) metabolic acidosis
(B) sulfisoxazole therapy
(C) hypoalbuminemia
(D) maternal ingestion of aspirin during pregnancy
— (E) maternal ingestion of phenobarbital during pregnancy

212. A 3-day-old infant is noted in the nursery to be jaundiced. Total serum bilirubin level is 10.5 mg per 100 ml (direct, 0.5 mg per 100 ml). Which of the following laboratory findings would be consistent with the diagnosis of physiologic jaundice in this infant?

(A) An elevated peripheral normoblast cell count
(B) An elevated level of hepatic glucuronyl transferase
(C) An elevated level of serum glutamic-oxaloacetic transaminase
(D) Normal excretion of Bromsulphalein
~ (E) None of the above

213. Which of the following conditions principally interferes with the mucosal phase of digestion?

(A) Zollinger-Ellison syndrome
(B) Enterokinase deficiency
—(C) *Giardia lamblia* infestation
(D) Gastrocolic fistula
(E) Biliary atresia

214. All the following statements concerning medium-chain triglycerides are true EXCEPT that

— (A) bile salts are required for their absorption
(B) they are incorporated into chylomicrons only to a minor degree
(C) during transport they are bound to albumin
(D) they are rapidly hydrolyzed by pancreatic lipase
(E) they are metabolized in the liver

215. A biopsy sample from the small intestine of a child is examined by light microscopy; a photomicrograph is shown below. The diagnosis most compatible with the findings depicted is

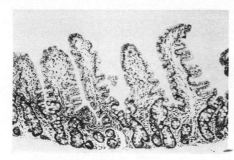

(A) celiac disease
(B) abetalipoproteinemia
(C) Whipple's disease
(D) congenital agammaglobulinemia
(E) sucrase-isomaltase deficiency

216. A child who has primary sucrase-isomaltase deficiency would be likely to have

(A) no family history of the disorder
(B) abnormal small-bowel mucosa
(C) reduced lactase activity
(D) reduced glucose absorption
(E) production of hydrogen following a sucrose load

217. The D-xylose tolerance test may be abnormal in individuals with any of the following conditions that are characterized by malabsorption EXCEPT

(A) celiac disease
(B) pancreatic deficiency
(C) bacterial overgrowth syndrome
(D) short bowel syndrome
(E) regional enteritis

218. Findings that are commonly associated with ulcerative colitis include

(A) rectal bleeding
(B) transmural pathology
(C) perianal abscesses
(D) "skip" lesions
(E) anorectal fistulas

219. Cirrhosis, complicated by portal hypertension, occurs in association with all the following disorders EXCEPT

(A) cystic fibrosis
(B) alpha$_1$-antitrypsin deficiency
(C) congenital hepatic fibrosis
(D) Wilson's disease
(E) histiocytosis X

220. A 3-week-old infant who is still at birth weight has bloody diarrhea. The child had delayed passage of meconium while in the newborn nursery. All the following disorders should be strongly considered in the differential diagnosis EXCEPT

(A) necrotizing enterocolitis
(B) cystic fibrosis
(C) Hirschsprung's disease
(D) hypothyroidism
(E) salmonellosis

221. A 3-year-old girl who has a prominent abdomen and lymphedema of the right arm is admitted to the hospital for investigation of her abdominal distension and persistent diarrhea. Initial laboratory findings include a total serum protein concentration of 3.2 g per 100 ml (albumin, 1.2 g per 100 ml). Based on these findings, the most likely diagnosis for this child would be

(A) Menetrier's disease
(B) cystic fibrosis
(C) tropical sprue
(D) intestinal lymphangiectasia
(E) severe pulmonic stenosis with heart failure

222. All the following are associated with hepatitis B EXCEPT

(A) chronic carrier state
(B) transmission from mother
(C) fulminant hepatitis
(D) live vaccine
(E) glomerulonephritis

223. Which of the following laboratory findings would be consistent with a diagnosis of Reye's syndrome?

(A) Hypoammonemia
(B) Cellular spinal fluid
(C) Leukopenia
(D) Diffusely abnormal electroencephalogram
(E) Shortened prothrombin time

224. A 6-week-old dehydrated child is admitted to a hospital following 10 days of vomiting. Pyloric stenosis is suspected. Which of the following findings would be most consistent with this diagnosis?

(A) Jaundice and indirect hyperbilirubinemia
(B) Hyponatremia with a hyperchloremic metabolic acidosis
(C) An elevated serum potassium level
(D) A urine specific gravity of 1.005
(E) A urine pH of 4.5

225. In a child who has long-standing cholestasis, the laboratory finding LEAST likely to be exhibited would be

(A) an elevated serum cholesterol level
(B) an elevated serum lipoprotein X level
(C) an elevated vitamin E concentration
(D) an elevated serum alkaline phosphatase level
(E) a normal prothrombin time

226. Which of the following is LEAST commonly associated with *Giardia lamblia*?

(A) Fecal-oral route
(B) Chronic carrier state
(C) Trophozoites and cysts in stool
(D) Tissue invasion
(E) Contaminated water

227. Which of the following clinical and pathologic findings is more characteristic of Crohn's disease than of ulcerative colitis?

(A) Rectal bleeding
(B) Short stature and delayed puberty
(C) Pericholangitis
(D) Toxic megacolon
(E) Small bowel involvement

228. Dietary fiber has been found to have which of the following relationships to irritable bowel syndrome, diverticular disease, colon cancer, obesity, and coronary artery disease?

(A) Increasing dietary fiber has been proven by controlled studies to decrease their incidence
(B) It has been suggested by epidemiological studies that increasing dietary fiber may lead to decrease in their incidence
(C) Dietary fiber levels have been shown to have no effect on any disease except constipation
(D) Increasing dietary fiber has been proven by controlled trials to increase their incidence
(E) Increasing dietary fiber has been shown to decrease their incidence, but only when given in infancy

229. All the following elements are considered to be valuable nutritional components of the child's diet EXCEPT

(A) zinc
(B) copper
(C) chromium
(D) lead
(E) molybdenum

230. The best long-term feeding for a 3-month-old infant in coma from head trauma is

(A) the standard hospital infant milk formula
(B) Alligator Ade
(C) Isoismo tube feeding
(D) apple juice
(E) Amphogel

231. When an infant with diarrhea has lost about 5 to 10 percent of his body weight over 2 days, all the following may be expected EXCEPT for

(A) depressed fontanel
(B) tachycardia
(C) moribund state
(D) sunken eyes
(E) loss of skin elasticity

232. Characteristics of hypernatremic dehydration with Na^+ in serum 170 mEq/L and 10 percent loss of body weight are all the following EXCEPT

(A) low blood pressure
(B) convulsions
(C) thirst
(D) lethargy
(E) hyperirritability

233. An acceptable solution for oral rehydration of infants with moderately severe diarrhea presumably caused by *E. coli* has the composition

(A) Na^+ 10 mEq/L, K^+ 15 mEq/L, Cl^- 25 mEq/L

(B) Na^+ 90 mEq/L, K^+ 15 mEq/L, Cl^- 75 mEq/L, HCO_3^- 30 mEq/L, glucose 111 mmol/L (2 g/100 ml)

(C) Na^+ 90 mEq/L, K^+ 15 mEq/L, Cl^- 75 mEq/L, HCO_3^- 30 mEq/L, glucose 333 mmol/L (6 g/100 ml)

(D) Na^+ 150 mEq/L, K^+ 15 mEq/L, Cl^- 135 mEq/L, HCO_3^- 30 mEq/L, glucose 111 mmol/L (2 g/100 ml)

(E) glucose 5 g/100 ml in isotonic saline (Na^+ 150 mEq/L, Cl^- 150 mEq/L)

DIRECTIONS: Each question below contains four suggested responses of which **one or more** is correct. Select

A	if	**1, 2, and 3**	are correct
B	if	**1 and 3**	are correct
C	if	**2 and 4**	are correct
D	if	**4**	is correct
E	if	**1, 2, 3, and 4**	are correct

234. Complications of parenteral nutrition include

(1) sepsis
(2) pulmonary emboli
(3) liver disease
(4) air emboli

235. Factors associated with human hepatitis B infection include which of the following?

(1) Oral-fecal transmission
(2) Dane particles
(3) Migratory arthritis
(4) Surface antigen

---

236. The x-ray shown below can suggest which of the following diagnoses?

(1) Chronic granulomatous disease
(2) Eosinophilic gastroenteritis
(3) Lymphoma
(4) Crohn's disease

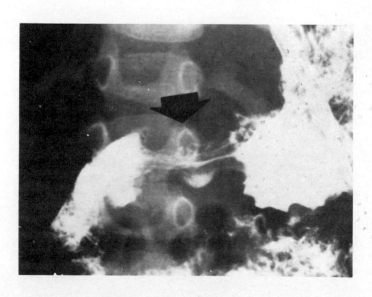

SUMMARY OF DIRECTIONS

A	B	C	D	E
1,2,3	1,3	2,4	4	All are
only	only	only	only	correct

237. Correct statements concerning Crohn's disease include

(1) it typically produces transmural lesions
(2) it can be associated with aphthous stomatitis in children
(3) it is associated with an increased incidence of colonic cancer
(4) it rarely spares the rectum

238. Gastrointestinal manifestations of cystic fibrosis include

(1) portal hypertension and varices
(2) an ileocecal mass
(3) abnormal gallbladder function
(4) intestinal obstruction

239. Disorders associated with disease of the terminal ileum include

(1) Crohn's disease
(2) Schönlein-Henoch purpura
(3) tuberculosis
(4) *Yersinia enterocolitica* infection

240. Correct statements about achalasia include which of the following?

(1) Lower esophageal sphincter pressure is elevated
(2) Lower esophageal sphincter fails to relax with swallowing
(3) It is associated with vagal and ganglionic degeneration
(4) It is usually associated with pseudoobstruction syndrome

241. Lactose intolerance can be diagnosed by which of the following laboratory studies?

(1) Blood glucose levels before and after oral administration of lactose
(2) Hydrogen excretion in breath after oral administration of lactose
(3) Stool pH and reducing substances
(4) Small intestinal biopsy and enzyme (lactase) assay

242. A 6-week-old infant is admitted to a hospital because of obstructive jaundice. Which of the following disorders could be responsible?

(1) Cystic fibrosis
(2) Gilbert's disease
(3) Alpha$_1$-antitrypsin deficiency
(4) Hypothyroidism

243. Conditions that are associated with abnormal function of the intestinal mucosa include which of the following?

(1) Dermatitis herpetiformis
(2) Hartnup disease
(3) Folic acid deficiency
(4) Cystic fibrosis

244. A 30-hour-old male infant, the product of a pregnancy complicated by polyhydramnios, presents with abdominal distension, poor feeding, and recurrent vomiting, the vomitus being bile stained. The infant has passed one meconium-stained stool. There is no evidence of fever, diarrhea, or melena. The physical examination is normal except for abdominal distension, mild jaundice, and hypotonic bowel sounds. A barium enema (see x-ray below) was obtained. A diagnostic and treatment regimen for this infant might include

(1) diatrizoate meglumine (Gastrografin) enemas
(2) small-bowel surgery
(3) pancreatic enzyme supplements
(4) rectal biopsy for ganglion cells

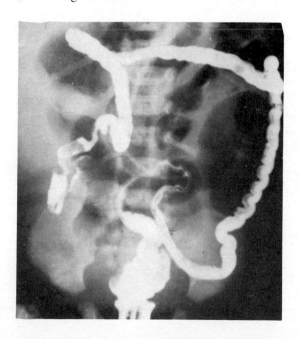

SUMMARY OF DIRECTIONS

A	B	C	D	E
1,2,3 only	1,3 only	2,4 only	4 only	All are correct

245. An 18-month-old girl was evaluated for poor growth during the prior
6 months, with iron deficiency anemia,
irritability, decrease in appetite, and
diarrhea. An upper gastrointestinal
series and small-bowel biopsy were
performed, the results of which are illustrated below. The possible pathogenic mechanisms operating in this
child include which of the following?

(1) Viral infection
—(2) Peptidase deficiency
(3) Endocrine disorder
—(4) Immunologic disorder

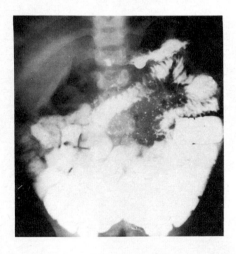 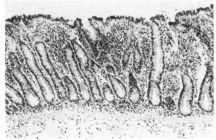

246. Kwashiorkor is characterized by

—(1) a history of inadequate protein intake with relatively adequate calories

(2) marked vulnerability to death from
intercurrent enteric infections

(3) edema

(4) hyperalbuminemia

DIRECTIONS: Each group of questions below consists of four lettered headings followed by a set of numbered items. For each numbered item select

A	if the item is associated with	(A) **only**
B	if the item is associated with	(B) **only**
C	if the item is associated with	**both** (A) and (B)
D	if the item is associated with	**neither** (A) nor (B)

Each lettered heading may be used **once, more than once, or not at all.**

Questions 247–251

(A) Non-A, non-B hepatitis
(B) Hepatitis B
(C) Both
(D) Neither

247. Currently the most common cause of transfusion-related hepatitis

248. Infectious agent is persistent in serum

249. Transmissible to an animal model

250. Chronic carrier state occurs

251. Vaccine to prevent the disease is available

Questions 252–256

(A) Wilson's disease
(B) Alpha$_1$-antitrypsin deficiency
(C) Both
(D) Neither

252. Symptoms often appear in the first year of life

253. Inherited as an autosomal recessive trait

254. Can be associated with pulmonary emphysema

255. Cause of postnecrotic cirrhosis

256. Can be associated with hemolytic episodes

Questions 257–262

(A) Total parenteral nutrition by central line
(B) Total parenteral nutrition by peripheral line
(C) Both
(D) Neither

257. Risk of bacterial and fungal sepsis

258. Thrombophlebitis of central veins

259. Superior vena cava obstruction syndrome occurs

260. Highly labor intensive for pediatric staff

261. Highly labor-intensive for nursing staff

262. Local damage to tissues may occur

DIRECTIONS: The group of questions below consists of lettered headings followed by a set of numbered items. For each numbered item select the **one** lettered heading with which it is **most** closely associated. Each lettered heading may be used **once, more than once, or not at all.**

Questions 263–267

For each description that follows, select the disorder with which it is most likely to be associated.

(A) Peutz-Jeghers syndrome
(B) Gardner's syndrome
(C) Juvenile polyps
(D) Juvenile polyposis of the colon
(E) Lymphoid polyposis

263. Commonly shows malignant degeneration

264. Is associated with soft-tissue masses

265. May be caused by *Giardia lamblia* infection

266. Is not inherited

267. Is associated with adenomatous polyps

The Gastrointestinal Tract

Answers

211. The answer is E. *(Silverman, ed 3. pp 19–21.)* Unconjugated bilirubin levels in serum above 20 mg per100 ml in full-term newborn infants can lead to diffusion of bilirubin into brain tissue and to neurologic damage. Sulfisoxazole and salicylates compete with bilirubin for binding sites on albumin; therefore, the presence of these drugs can cause dislocation of bilirubin to tissues. Metabolic acidosis also reduces binding of bilirubin. Administration of phenobarbital has been used to induce glucuronyl transferase in newborn infants and thus can reduce, rather than exacerbate, neonatal jaundice.

212. The answer is E. *(Behrman, ed 12. pp 378–380.)* A transient elevation of unconjugated bilirubin levels in serum is commonly found in newborn infants (physiologic jaundice or hyperbilirubinemia of the newborn). Aside from an elevation in serum bilirubin levels, infants who have physiologic jaundice typically demonstrate normal laboratory findings. In full-term infants, liver function studies are normal. Defects in coagulation are not observed, and complete blood cell counts are within normal limits. Examination of urine would not show the presence of bile. Tests such as Bromsulphalein excretion study, which evaluates conjugation, would be prolonged.

213. The answer is C. *(Silverman, ed 3. pp 262–265.)* The intraluminal phase of digestion involves the hydrolysis and solubilization of fats, proteins, and complex carbohydrates. Acid hypersecretion in individuals who have Zollinger-Ellison syndrome results in the inactivation of pancreatic enzymes and the precipitation of bile salts. Enterokinase deficiency restricts the activation of trypsin. Biliary atresia prevents the excretion of bile salts, and a gastrocolic fistula can lead to bacterial overgrowth in the small intestine. Unlike these disorders, which interfere with the intraluminal phase of digestion, infestation by *Giardia lamblia* causes malabsorption by damaging the intestinal mucosa.

214. The answer is A. *(Greenberger, N Engl J Med 280:1047, 1969.)* Medium-chain triglycerides consist of fatty acids that contain from 8 to 12 carbon atoms and bypass the usual mucosal pathway of triglyceride resynthesis. They are rapidly hydrolyzed by pancreatic lipase; and because the fatty acids and monoglycerides are water soluble, bile salts are not necessary. Medium-chain triglycerides are transported (albumin-bound) principally in the portal blood; in the liver they undergo nearly complete metabolism.

215. The answer is E. *(Silverman, ed 3. pp 242–243. Trier, N Engl J Med 285: 1470, 1973.)* When examined by light microscopy, a biopsy sample from the small intestine of an individual who has sucrase-isomaltase deficiency will appear normal. In the other disorders listed in the question, however, histologic examination of the small bowel reveals the presence of diagnostic or at least highly characteristic lesions. In sucrase-isomaltase deficiency, analysis of the intestinal disaccharidase enzymes demonstrates normal lactase activity with an absence of the sucrase enzyme. Therapy should include removal of the offending sugar from the diet.

216. The answer is E. *(Silverman, ed 3. pp 242–243.)* Sucrase-isomaltase deficiency is an inherited autosomal recessive condition characterized by a reduction in or absence of this disaccharidase. As in other disaccharidase deficiencies, such as lactase deficiency, intestinal mucosa is normal on histologic examination of a biopsy sample. Malabsorption of sucrose results in bacterial metabolism of carbohydrate and production of hydrogen. The mechanism of glucose absorption is independent of—and thus unaffected by a deficiency in—sucrase-isomaltase activity.

217. The answer is B. *(Silverman, ed 3. pp 894–895.)* D-Xylose absorption is a measure of mucosal function of the small intestine. Diseases such as gluten-induced enteropathy (celiac disease) and regional enteritis that damage small bowel intestinal mucosa will cause abnormal D-xylose absorption values. Because pancreatic insufficiency disrupts the intraluminal phase of digestion, the mucosal transport is not altered. Patients with short bowel syndrome have decreased absorption owing to decreased absorptive surface area.

218. The answer is A. *(Braunwald, ed 11. pp 1277–1287. Sleisenger, ed 3. pp 1122–1164.)* Ulcerative colitis characteristically is associated with a continuous lesion involving the superficial mucosal tissue of the colon. Rectal bleeding and, especially, bloody diarrhea are major symptoms; however, the severity of the symptoms, the clinical course, and the prognosis are highly variable. Sigmoidoscopic examination typically shows increased mucosal friability and decreased mucosal detail. Anorectal fistulas and perianal abscesses are much more common in individuals who have Crohn's disease. Extraintestinal manifestations, such as skin lesions and liver disease, are not uncommon in association with ulcerative colitis.

219. The answer is C. *(Kerr, Q J Med 30:91–117, 1961. Silverman, ed 3. p 738.)* All the conditions listed in the question are associated with portal hypertension, and all but congenital hepatic fibrosis are associated with cirrhosis as well. Children who have congenital hepatic fibrosis usually present with portal hypertension and upper gastrointestinal bleeding; their portal hypertension is due to a presinusoidal block, and they have normal liver function. The findings of associated renal lesions and a positive family history help confirm the diagnosis of congenital hepatic fibrosis. In the other disorders listed in the question, liver disease is a primary or associated finding that can be complicated by cirrhosis.

220. The answer is D. *(Schapiro, pp 217–236. Silverman, ed 3. pp 69–70.)* Delayed passage of meconium occurs in a high percentage of children who have Hirschsprung's disease. These children may develop enterocolitic complications, poor weight gain, and diarrhea—rather than constipation—in the first few months of life. Infections including salmonellosis may cause bloody diarrhea in a neonate and occur frequently in association with Hirschsprung's disease. Dilatation, necrosis, perforation, and intramural pneumatosis of the ileum and colon, often with bloody diarrhea, are characteristics of necrotizing enterocolitis, an idiopathic complication of prematurity, exchange transfusions, and severe neonatal infection. Other conditions associated with delayed passage of meconium include a meconium plug, inspissated meconium accompanying cystic fibrosis, and hypothyroidism. An infant who has hypothyroidism, however, usually is constipated; diarrhea rarely occurs in association with this disorder.

221. The answer is D. *(Silverman, ed 3. pp 308–312.)* The child described in the question has abnormally low levels of serum albumin and total serum protein. Intestinal lymphangiectasia is a type of protein-losing enteropathy that probably results from a congenital abnormality of the lymphatic system. It is frequently associated with chronic lymphatic obstruction and lymphedema in various parts of the body, such as the hands, the arms, and especially the legs. Children who have intestinal lymphangiectasia have hypoproteinemia as a result of protein loss from the small bowel. These children also have lymphocytopenia. Other associated findings include abnormal delayed hypersensitivity, hypocalcemia, malabsorption, edema, and occasionally pleural effusions. Treatment with a low-fat diet, supplemented by medium-chain triglycerides, often reduces lymph flow and may be beneficial. Although severe right-sided heart disease and Menetrier's disease both may cause protein loss in the gastrointestinal tract, they rarely are associated with lymphatic aberrations. Diarrhea and growth problems are common to tropical sprue and cystic fibrosis, both of which also can lead to protein loss from the bowel.

222. The answer is D. *(Silverman, ed 3. pp 580–600.)* Hepatitis B infection may result in a chronic carrier state and is transmitted from mother to infant. Fulminant hepatitis and glomerulonephritis secondary to immune complex deposition are recognized complications. Vaccination with good immunity is achieved using a killed inactivated vaccine that does not contain live virus.

223. The answer is D. *(Braunwald, ed 11. p 1354. Partin, N Engl J Med 285:1139–1143, 1971. Reye, Lancet 2:749–757, 1963. Silverman, ed 3. pp 630–653.)*

Reye's syndrome usually begins as a mild, nonspecific viral illness that worsens suddenly, possibly in relation to taking aspirin, and leads to encephalopathy and hepatic dysfunction. Specific biochemical deficiencies, including deficiency of ornithine transcarbamylase, have been suggested. The urea cycle does not seem to be primarily involved. Serum levels of ammonia, amino acids, and glutamic-oxaloacetic transaminase are elevated in affected children; white blood cell count also is higher than normal. Other laboratory findings include hypoglycemia, prolonged prothrombin time, and acellular cerebrospinal fluid. Mitochondrial lesions predominate in the brain and liver; and, in the proper clinical setting, microvesicular hepatic steatosis is diagnostic for the disorder. Electroencephalographic examination is diffusely abnormal and typically demonstrates high-voltage, slow-wave activity.

224. The answer is A. *(Scharli, J Pediatr Surg 4:108–114, 1969.)* Symptoms and signs of pyloric stenosis include vomiting, dehydration, constipation, moderate jaundice (indirect hyperbilirubinemia), and a palpable mass in the right upper quadrant. The differential diagnosis, particularly in male infants, should include salt loss caused by one type of the adrenogenital syndrome; infants with this disorder characteristically are acidotic and have an elevated serum potassium level. In contrast, infants who have pyloric stenosis have metabolic alkalosis and an alkaline, concentrated urine.

225. The answer is C. *(Guggenheim, J Pediatr 100:51–58, 1982.)* Absorption of vitamin E, a lipovitamin, is decreased in children with long-standing cholestasis. The deficiency state is occasionally associated with a sensory neuropathy, optic degeneration, and deficiency of upward gaze. Vitamin E levels must be correlated with total serum lipids when evaluating the deficiency state. Obstructive liver disease causes elevation of serum cholesterol and alkaline phosphatase levels; the serum level of lipoprotein X, an abnormal lipoprotein that accumulates in the absence of proper amounts of lecithin-cholesterol acyltransferase, also is increased. Although prothrombin time is vitamin K sensitive, it often remains normal until deficiency of this lipid-soluble vitamin becomes severe.

226. The answer is D. *(Sleisenger, ed 3. pp 986–989.)* Giardia lamblia, the first protozoan parasite to be described, is a common parasitic infestation. It is acquired by ingestion of cysts acquired from contaminated drinking water, with known reservoirs being dogs and beavers. Fecal-oral contamination is reported to occur. Mechanisms for pathogenesis are not certain, although epithelial damage and secondary dissacharide deficiencies have been documented. Clinical features include prolonged diarrhea and signs of malabsorption such as flatulence, weight loss, and failure to thrive. A chronic carrier state occurs, often in patients with immunodeficiency or hypogammaglobulinemia. Tissue invasion is uncommon. Treatment agents include quinacrine, metronidazole, and tinidazole.

227. The answer is E. *(Behrman, ed 12. pp 921–925. Silverman, ed 3. pp 337–389. Sleisenger, ed 3. pp 1088–1118.)* Small bowel involvement differentiates ulcerative colitis from Crohn's disease: in the latter any area of the small intestinal tract and colon may be affected, whereas in ulcerative colitis only the colon is involved. Growth failure and delayed puberty may occur in both conditions but are more common in Crohn's disease, often presenting in an insidious fashion. Rectal friability and bleeding are commonly associated with both ulcerative colitis and Crohn's disease, whereas toxic megacolon and pericholangitis are more often complications of ulcerative colitis. Isolated small bowel disease should be differentiated from lymphoma or infection by the appropriate diagnostic procedures before assuming Crohn's disease as the etiology.

228. The answer is B. *(Forbes, ed 2. pp 99–103.)* Epidemiological studies have indicated the possibility that increasing dietary fiber will decrease the incidence of the diseases listed in the question by increasing stool bulk and decreasing transit time through the intestines. Dietary fiber affects the metabolism of a variety of nutrients so that firm recommendations for the nutrition of infants and children cannot be made at this time. It is probably not needed in the diet of infants under the age of 1 year.

229. The answer is D. *(Forbes, ed 2. p 740.)* Lead has no known role in human nutrition and is a toxin with no known lower limit of normal levels. The others listed are trace elements that are vital components of enzyme systems. Zinc, copper, chromium, and molybdenum are provided in the diet by meat.

230. The answer is A. *(Forbes, ed 2. pp 358–362.)* Information is lacking on the suitability of commercially prepared tube feedings for use in infants and children under 4 years of age. The standard for comparison is the infant formula, which is easily administered by tube. The percentage of calories from protein from some of the tube feedings is excessive for infants and some may require supplementation with vitamin D, calcium, and iron.

231. The answer is C. *(Finberg, p 118.)* A moribund state is characteristic of a loss of about 15 percent of body weight from dehydration. The other findings are characteristic of a loss of body weight of 5 to 10 percent when there is no hypernatremia. Additional findings at this level of dehydration may be coolness and acrocyanosis of the extremities and poor heart sounds, but blood pressure is usually maintained in the normal range.

232. The answer is A. *(Finberg, pp 80–81.)* The extracellular fluid and circulating blood volumes tend to be preserved with hypernatremic dehydration, at the expense of the intracellular volume. Therefore, hypotension is not characteristic nor are the other signs of circulatory inadequacy that are typical of isotonic or hypotonic dehydration. Signs suggesting involvement of the central nervous system are characteristic of hypertonic dehydration.

233. The answer is B. *(Finberg, pp 152–154.)* The solution outlined in B has the actual composition of the oral rehydration solution recommended by the World Health Organization. The glucose concentrations in solutions C and E are too high and may cause osmotic diarrhea in some patients. The sodium concentrations of solutions D and E are too high for continuing use beyond the first few hours of deficit correction because hypernatremia would develop. The sodium composition of solution A is too low to replace losses and hyponatremia would develop.

234. The answer is E (all). *(Finberg, pp 141–145, 230–232. Forbes, ed 2. pp 155–156.)* Parenteral nutrition, particularly when using a central line, has a relatively high risk of complications so that it should not be used without good indication. In addition to the complications mentioned, thrombosis of central veins, perforations of veins with infusion and bleeding into the pleural space and other sites, pneumothorax, brachial plexus injury, and skin sloughing may also occur. Awareness of these complications and the practice of careful techniques may minimize the risks of this sometimes lifesaving nutritional procedure.

235. The answer is E (all). *(Alpert, N Engl J Med 285:185–189, 1971. Sabesin, N Engl J Med 290:944–950, 996–1002, 1974.)* Human hepatitis B (serum hepatitis) is associated with the hepatitis B antigen and can be identified by the presence of surface antigens, core antigens, or Dane particles, which are thought to be intact hepatitis B viruses. A prodrome of migratory arthritis or skin rash recently has been recognized and presumably is due to surface antigen-antibody immune complexes. Although traditionally associated with hepatitis A, oral-fecal transmission also has been linked to hepatitis B.

236. The answer is E (all). *(Greseon, Pediatrics 54:456, 1974. Sleisenger, ed 3. pp 162–185.)* The x-ray presented in the question shows antral narrowing, an unusual finding in children. This finding should not be considered as indicating only an ulcer, as it can be associated with all the disorders listed in the question. Hence, the confirmed diagnosis of these conditions cannot be made on the basis of x-ray alone. A per oral gastric biopsy is necessary in order to differentiate one from the other.

237. The answer is A (1,2,3). *(Braunwald, ed 11. pp 1277–1287. Silverman, ed 3. pp 370–389.)* Crohn's disease (granulomatous colitis) characteristically is associated with transmural, granulomatous intestinal lesions that are discontinuous and can appear in both the small and large intestine. Although Crohn's disease first may appear as a rectal fissure or fistula, the rectum often is spared. Aphthous stomatitis is a common complaint in affected children. In relation to the general population, the risk of colonic carcinoma in affected individuals is increased but not nearly to the degree associated with ulcerative colitis.

238. The answer is E (all). *(Silverman, ed 3. pp 819–832. Sleisenger, ed 3. pp 1436–1450.)* Children who have cystic fibrosis can exhibit a wide range of gastrointestinal disorders: indeed, malabsorption in children is more likely to be due to cystic fibrosis than to any other cause. Hepatic lesions associated with cystic fibrosis include portal hypertension (often accompanied by varices and ascites), cirrhosis, and fatty disease. Among affected newborn infants, meconium ileus occurs. Obstruction in older children can occur for a variety of reasons. Gallbladder disorders associated with cystic fibrosis include congenital microgallbladder and cholelithiasis.

239. The answer is E (all). *(Silverman, ed 3. pp 347, 375, 389.)* Crohn's disease is a granulomatous disorder that can affect any area of the small or large intestine; another granulomatous disorder, tuberculosis, can lead to ileocecal disease. Intestinal lesions of Schönlein-Henoch purpura can be caused by hemorrhage into the mucosal wall; almost any area of the gastrointestinal tract, however, can be similarly affected. *Yersinia enterocolitica* infection causes an acute gastroenteritis or a more persistent, localized disease involving the colon and distal ileum, often mimicking inflammatory bowel disease.

240. The answer is A (1, 2, 3). *(Silverman, ed 3. pp 158–161.)* Esophageal achalasia is a disease of unknown etiology characterized by the absence of peristalsis in the body of the esophagus and by failure of the lower esophageal sphincter (LES) to relax in response to swallowing. Histologically, there is degeneration of Auerbach's plexus and intraneural nerve cells. Motility patterns reveal elevated lower esophageal pressure with a failure to initiate neural relaxation of LES in response to swallowing. This should be differentiated from organic strictures of the lower esophagus. This disease is not associated with pseudoobstruction syndrome, which involves motor disorders of the small and large intestine as well as the esophagus.

241. The answer is E (all). *(Braunwald, ed 11. p 1274. Silverman, ed 3. pp 14, 15, 300, 888–897.)* Lactase is a disaccharidase localized in the brush border of the intestinal villous cells. It hydrolyzes lactose to its constituent monosaccharides, glucose and galactose. Intestinal lactase levels are usually normal at birth in all populations; however, lactase deficiency is a common genetically predetermined condition with an incidence reported to be 5 to 15 percent of the adult white population and 80 to 90 percent of adult blacks and Asians. Sucrose, also a disaccharide, is a nonreducing sugar composed of glucose and fructose that is hydrolyzed by the brush border enzyme sucrase. Lactase activity is not readily increased by the oral administration of substrate or the inclusion of lactose in the diet. The clinical symptoms of lactose malabsorption are due to the presence of osmotically active, undigested lactose, which may act to increase intestinal fluid volume, alter transit time, and produce the symptoms of abdominal cramps, distension, and, occasionally, watery diarrhea. Bacterial metabolism of the nonabsorbed carbohydrates in the colon to carbon dioxide and hydrogen may contribute to the clinical symptoms. Acquired lactase deficiency is often associated with conditions of the gastrointestinal tract that cause intestinal mucosal injury (e.g., sprue and regional enteritis).

Diagnostic techniques for lactose intolerance include removal of the offending sugar with a reproduction of symptoms following an oral load (2 g/kg, maximum 50 g) accompanied by failure of blood sugar to rise more than 30 mg per 100 ml. Although the ingestion of even small amounts of lactose can be diagnostic if gastrointestinal symptoms occur, the measurement of breath hydrogen is more specific as it is not affected by glucose metabolism or gastric emptying. Similarly, an acidic stool pH in the presence of reducing substances would be diagnostic. Direct measurement of enzyme levels combined with histologic evaluation helps to differentiate an acquired (secondary versus primary) lactase deficiency in which the intestinal histology is normal.

242. The answer is B (1, 3). (*Silverman, ed 3. pp 21, 494–555.*) Obstructive jaundice (i.e., a direct-reacting bilirubin greater than 15 percent of the total) requires investigation in all infants. Cystic fibrosis and alpha$_1$-antitrypsin deficiency should be considered in the diagnostic evaluation of any child with these presenting findings. Other diseases to be excluded include galactosemia, tyrosinemia, and urinary tract or other infections, including toxoplasmosis, cytomegalovirus, rubella, syphilis, and herpesvirus. Ultrasound examination to rule out choledochus cyst may be included with an ^{131}I rose bengal or ^{99}technetium hepatic imindodiacetic acid (HIDA) scan to assess the patency of the biliary tree. Liver biopsy may show evidence of hepatitis and giant cell transformation both in cystic fibrosis and alpha$_1$-antitrypsin deficiency. These findings may differentiate these diseases from extrahepatic obstruction or biliary atresia, but they are not pathognomonic in themselves. The presence of diastase-resistant, periodic acid Schiff (PAS)–positive granules is reported but is not specific in alpha$_1$-antitrypsin deficiency alone. In contrast, infants who have Gilbert's syndrome or hypothyroidism present with an indirect hyperbilirubinemia and have normal liver biopsies.

243. The answer is A (1, 2, 3). (*Silverman, ed 3. pp 265–279.*) Hartnup disease, folic acid deficiency, and dermatitis herpetiformis are all associated with abnormal function of the intestinal mucosa. Hartnup disease is an inborn defect in the absorption by intestinal epithelial cells of the amino acid tryptophan. Folate deficiency, either from a congenital disorder or in association with the malabsorption syndrome, signals jejunal mucosal dysfunction. Dermatitis herpetiformis may be associated with fat malabsorption. Cystic fibrosis interferes with the intraluminal phase of digestion.

244. The answer is A (1, 2, 3). (*Silverman, ed 3. pp 814–835.*) The x-ray presented in the question shows a microcolon (disuse microcolon), which is characteristic of fetal intestinal obstruction; it requires prompt diagnosis and therapeutic management. Films of the abdomen are the first step in establishing the diagnosis and possible level of obstruction in an infant with abdominal distension and clinical evidence of obstruction. With meconium ileus or meconium peritonitis a character-istic "soap bubble" appearance in the right lower quadrant or evidence of intestinal perforation might be evident. Barium enema is then often required to establish the presence of microcolon and to differentiate between a volvulus and other less com-mon abnormalities. Ileal atresia, intestinal perforation, and meconium peritonitis are frequently associated with cystic fibrosis. These begin in utero and are accompanied by a secondary microcolon. Occasionally, a microcolon may be present when acute intestinal obstruction caused by malrotation and volvulus occurs very early in life. Evidence by barium enema of abnormal placement or lack of fixation of the cecum can suggest this diagnosis. Obstruction in Down's syndrome (trisomy 21) infants also can be caused by jejunoileal atresia, which may be accompanied by malrotation.

Tracheoesophageal fistula with esophageal atresia is associated with polyhy-dramnios. It does not lead to microcolon unless there is complete obstruction. Hirsch-sprung's disease presents in the newborn period with delayed passage of meconium but with a normal or increased diameter of the colon; occasionally, there is evidence of enterocolitis. A transition zone may be seen by barium enema, often with failure to clear the barium over the next 24 hours.

Surgery is usually required to correct meconium ileus. However, occasionally a diatrizoate meglumine (Gastrografin) or N-acetylcysteine (5 to 10% solution) enema has relieved the obstruction. Enzyme replacement is required in the therapy of the pancreatic insufficiency associated with the cystic fibrosis of this patient with me-conium ileus.

245. The answer is C (2, 4). *(Behrman, ed 12. 933–934. Silverman, ed 3. p 272.)* Symptoms of celiac disease, which include chronic vomiting and diarrhea, irritabil-ity, and failure to grow, most commonly present during the first 2 years of life. Small bowel x-rays of affected children often show thickened and coarse mucosal folds and dilatation of the intestine; small-bowel biopsy can show severely abnormal morphology. Celiac disease, an inherited condition in which the symptoms of mal-absorption may occur sporadically within a family, is characterized by an intolerance to gluten. Treatment of affected children with a gluten-free diet is effective; however, removal of the offending agent is insufficient to establish the diagnosis. Histological recovery after removal of gluten is required, and on occasion it may be necessary to demonstrate recurrence of injury with gluten challenge. Proposed mechanisms for the initiation of injury include the absence of an intracellular or brush border pep-tidase, which renders the individual unable to digest gluten, and an immunologically mediated mechanism that involves the recognition of gluten as an offending agent. Histological features include an abnormal surface epithelium with loss of columnar cells, shortened villi, and elongation of crypts. While these are not specific for gluten-sensitive enteropathy, they are histologically consistent. Granuloma formation is not seen in celiac disease, nor is a pronounced eosinophilic inflammatory com-ponent. Treatment always involves gluten withdrawal and may also include a lactose-free diet if sufficient mucosal damage has occurred. Corticosteroids are reserved for use in acute celiac crises and in supportive management.

The histopathology of some other diarrheal diseases is as follows: ulcerative colitis does not involve the small intestine, and the small-bowel biopsy in cystic fibrosis is normal. In lymphangiectasia the biopsy shows dilated lymphatics with a normal mucosa. In primary agammaglobulinemia there is an absence of plasma cells and a variety of histological abnormalities, particularly when complicated by giardiasis, malnutrition, or both. In congenital lactase deficiency, the small-bowel biopsy is normal, and the diagnosis is established by enzyme analysis.

246. The answer is A (1,2,3). *(Finberg, pp 158–162.)* In kwashiorkor dietary protein deficiency, after weaning, leads to low serum albumin causing decreased plasma volume and increased interstitial fluid or edema. If there is marked caloric deficit, marasmus occurs. These patients have a high death rate from intercurrent infections.

247–251. The answers are: 247-A, 248-C, 249-C, 250-C, 251-B. *(Rudolph, ed 17. pp 616–620.)* Non-A, non-B hepatitis is now the most common cause of post-transfusion hepatitis since the advent of sensitive screening methods for hepatitis B surface antigen in transfused blood. Current estimates for the prevalence of non-A, non-B hepatitis as a cause of transfusion-related hepatitis range between 50 to 90 percent. Persistence of infectious agents has been documented in both diseases. They are both transmissible to animals. A chronic carrier state occurs with both non-A, non-B hepatitis and hepatitis B. Recent studies have demonstrated the efficacy and safety of a vaccine for hepatitis B; however, no vaccine is available for non-A, non-B hepatitis at the current time, nor has an identifiable agent(s) been isolated.

252–256. The answers are: 252-B, 253-A, 254-B, 255-C, 256-A. *(Silverman, ed 3. pp 700–711, 714–716.)* Wilson's disease, an autosomal recessive genetic disorder, is characterized by the defective metabolism of copper. Copper deposition particularly affects the brain—causing tremors, dystonia, and personality changes—and the liver—causing portal hypertension and postnecrotic cirrhosis among other conditions. Hemolysis can lead to recurrent jaundice and anemia. Renal defects, which are associated with glycosuria and aminoaciduria, often occur. Wilson's disease usually appears clinically in individuals between the ages of 6 and 20 years. Administration of D-penicillamine has been therapeutically helpful.

Alpha₁-antitrypsin deficiency, which has an autosomal codominant mode of inheritance, can cause chronic liver disease in infants and may give rise in adults to gradually developing dyspnea as a result of panacinar emphysema, early symptoms of which can appear in childhood. Jaundice can develop in affected infants during the first weeks of life; histological examination of the liver shows intralobular bile stasis, perilobular fibrosis, and other abnormalities. Postnecrotic cirrhosis develops later. Management includes symptomatic treatment and genetic counseling.

257–262. The answers are: 257-C, 258-A, 259-A, 260-B, 261-C, 262-C. *(Finberg, pp 141–145, 230–232.)* Owing to the risks of complications, some of which are listed here, total parenteral nutrition should not be instituted or continued without good justification. The enteral route, when available, is almost always preferable. Pediatric staff in intensive care units find it much less work for them to have the surgeons put in a central line than to have to constantly monitor and replace peripheral lines. There is, therefore, a drift toward central, total parenteral nutrition, even though some of its hazards to the patient are greater. Skin sloughs are more likely with peripheral lines, but central lines may perforate central vessels and allow bleeding and infusion of irritating or toxic material into deeper tissues or the pleural space. Both types of infusions have a substantial risk of bacterial and fungal sepsis. Use of central lines permits damaging infusion of concentrated solutions directly into the heart, brain, or liver if the tip of the catheter is misplaced. Another complication of central lines is thrombosis of central veins, which can have severe long-term consequences, including superior vena cava obstruction syndrome.

263–267. The answers are: 263-B, 264-B, 265-E, 266-C, 267-B. *(Silverman, ed 3. pp 455–465.)* All the disorders listed have gastrointestinal polyposis. Peutz-Jeghers syndrome, which is inherited as an autosomal dominant trait, is characterized by the presence of hamartomatous polyps, especially in the small intestine but also occasionally in the stomach and colon. The most striking extraintestinal manifestation of this disorder is lip or buccal pigmentation, which usually develops during infancy. Peutz-Jeghers polyposis rarely leads to carcinoma.

Gardner's syndrome, on the other hand, is characterized by adenomatous polyps that frequently undergo malignant degeneration. This autosomal dominant disorder occurs mainly in the colon, but may also involve the small intestine. In affected children under the age of 10 years, the condition may appear first as a fibromatous mass or epidermoid cyst involving skin or soft tissue.

Isolated juvenile polyps occur as a benign, nonheritable condition typically associated with pedunculated inflammatory polyps that usually occur within 25 cm of the anus. Juvenile polyposis of the colon, in contrast, is an inherited condition (the mode of inheritance is unknown) causing large numbers of juvenile polyps to appear in the intestine. Neither disorder is associated with malignant degeneration. Although children having juvenile polyposis of the colon may have other congenital anomalies, children with juvenile polyps usually do not.

Lymphoid polyposis (nodular lymphoid hyperplasia) can affect both the small and the large intestine. In cases where the appearance of the submucosal nodules, which are composed of lymphoid follicles, is confined to the small intestine, infection with *Giardia lamblia* may be an etiologic factor. Lymphoid polyposis is associated neither with intestinal carcinoma nor with extraintestinal manifestations. Whether this condition is inherited is not known.

The Urinary Tract

DIRECTIONS: Each question below contains five suggested responses. Select the **one best** response to each question.

268. The presence of drug-induced nephrotic syndrome should be most highly suspected in a proteinuric patient who has received which of the following drugs?

(A) Tetracycline
(B) Streptomycin
— (C) Trimethadione
(D) Diazepam
(E) Chlorambucil

269. An *Escherichia coli* colony count of 2000/mm³ would be definite evidence of a urinary tract infection if the sampled urine

(A) has a specific gravity of 1.008
(B) has been taken from a catheterized bladder and has a specific gravity of 1.022
(C) is from an ileal-loop bag
— (D) is from a suprapubic tap
(E) is the first morning sample

270. A renal biopsy is performed on a 10-year-old boy with hematuria and proteinuria; a micrograph from the biopsy is shown below. The most likely diagnosis is

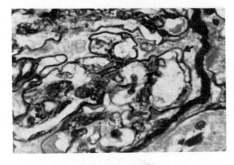

(A) segmental glomerulosclerosis
(B) postinfectious glomerulonephritis
— (C) membranoproliferative glomerulonephritis
(D) crescentic glomerulonephritis
(E) focal global glomerulosclerosis

271. An 8-year-old girl has a glomerular filtration rate of 100 ml/min per 1.73 m². Her urine specific gravity does not exceed 1.010. These laboratory values could be associated with all the following conditions EXCEPT

(A) diabetes insipidus
(B) sickle cell anemia
— (C) childhood nephrosis
(D) nephrocalcinosis
(E) pyelonephritis

272. The cells shown below were seen on microscopic examination of a bacteriologically sterile urine specimen. The differential diagnosis should include all the following conditions EXCEPT

(A) renal tuberculosis
(B) systemic lupus erythematosus
(C) interstitial nephritis
—(D) Potter's syndrome
(E) Kawasaki disease

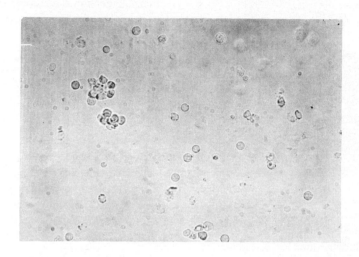

273. A blood pressure of 120/80 mm Hg is elevated for children aged

—(A) 4 years
(B) 7 years
—(C) 10 years
(D) 12 years
(E) 15 years

274. An exogenous substance that is used to measure glomerular filtration rate should be

(A) physiologically active
(B) capable of binding with plasma proteins
—(C) freely filterable at the glomerulus
(D) secreted by the renal tubule
(E) reabsorbed by the renal tubule

275. The child shown in the photograph below most likely has

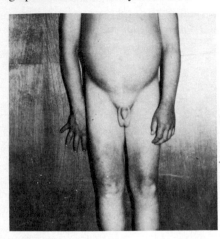

(A) cystinosis
(B) polycystic kidneys
(C) diabetes insipidus
(D) acute poststreptococcal glomerulonephritis
(E) nephrosis

276. A 7-year-old boy suffers multiple injuries as a result of blunt abdominal trauma. All the following statements concerning the proper assessment and treatment of the injuries are true EXCEPT that

(A) most renal injuries can be managed nonoperatively
(B) major vascular injuries require rapid surgical intervention
(C) rupture of a full bladder is impossible
(D) traumatic hematocele requires surgical exploration and repair
(E) prompt surgical repair is needed for most ureteral injuries

277. A 3-year-old boy develops edema and proteinuria. His serum cholesterol level is 322 mg per 100 ml, and his serum albumin level is 1.9 g per 100 ml. The likelihood that he has minimal-change nephrotic syndrome is about

(A) 10 percent
(B) 25 percent
(C) 40 percent
(D) 65 percent
(E) 80 percent

278. Funduscopic examination of a 13-year-old girl shows general and focal arteriolar narrowing. A hemorrhage is observed in the left retina, and sclerosis is present. Her blood pressure is 180/110 mm Hg. This girl would be likely to exhibit all the following symptoms or signs EXCEPT

(A) isolated facial nerve palsy
(B) headache
(C) hyporeflexia
(D) nocturnal wakening
(E) left ventricular hypertrophy

279. A 10-month-old child has diarrhea and has lost about 10 percent of her body weight. Laboratory analysis reveals a serum sodium level of 162 mEq/L. The clinical sign or symptom that would be LEAST likely to accompany these findings would be

(A) increased reflexes
(B) impaired mental status
(C) marked thirst
(D) marked loss of circulatory volume
(E) doughy skin

280. The photomicrograph shown below of a urine specimen from a 7-year-old child is LEAST likely to support a diagnosis of

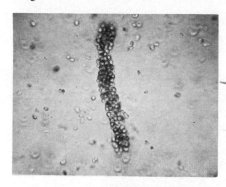

(A) systemic lupus erythematosus
(B) acute poststreptococcal glomerulonephritis
(C) Berger disease
—(D) membranous glomerulopathy
(E) mesangiocapillary glomerulonephritis

281. During the first year of a child's life, all the following increase EXCEPT

(A) glomerular filtration rate
— (B) nephron number
(C) renal plasma flow
(D) tubular reabsorptive capacity
(E) tubular secretory capacity

282. A 7-year-old boy has crampy abdominal pain and a rash on the back of his legs and buttocks as well as on the extensor surfaces of his forearms. Laboratory analysis reveals proteinuria and microhematuria. He is most likely to be affected by

(A) systemic lupus erythematosus
—(B) anaphylactoid purpura
(C) poststreptococcal glomerulonephritis
(D) polyarteritis nodosa
(E) dermatomyositis

283. Ingestion of which of the following products should be treated by the administration of ethanol?

—(A) antifreeze
(B) chalk
(C) hand lotion
(D) Vaseline
(E) lipstick

DIRECTIONS: Each question below contains four suggested responses of which
one or more is correct. Select

A	if	**1, 2, and 3**	are correct
B	if	**1 and 3**	are correct
C	if	**2 and 4**	are correct
D	if	**4**	is correct
E	if	**1, 2, 3, and 4**	are correct

284. The angiogram below is from a
12-year-old boy who has large kidneys.
Findings on the x-ray are consistent
with

(1) multicystic renal dysplasia
(2) nephronophthisis
(3) megacalyx
(4) adult-type polycystic disease

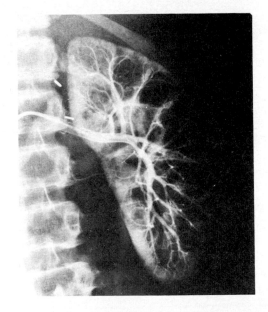

285. Correct statements concerning nephrogenic diabetes insipidus include which of the following?

(1) Most North American patients are of common descent
(2) It is probably inherited by an X-linked recessive mode
(3) It is a likely consequence of an enzymatic or biochemical renal tubular abnormality
(4) It is usually diagnosed at birth

286. Patients with shunt nephritis typically have

(1) red blood cell casts in the urine
(2) decreased C3 level in serum
(3) hypertension
(4) positive urine culture for bacteria

287. The onset of chronic renal failure is likely to be associated with which of the following findings?

(1) Growth retardation
(2) Oliguria
(3) Anorexia
(4) Hypotonia

288. The findings one might expect in a 6-year-old boy with brown urine and healing impetigo include which of the following?

(1) Hypertension
(2) Dyspnea
(3) Periorbital edema
(4) Hepatomegaly

289. An arteriogram of an 8-year-old girl who has hypertension is shown below. Findings illustrated in the arteriogram could be the result of

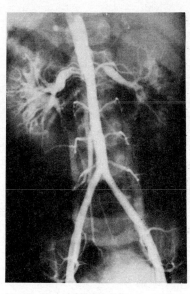

(1) fibromuscular dysplasia
(2) von Recklinghausen's disease
(3) tumorous impingement
(4) arteriovenous malformation

290. An 11-year-old girl repeatedly has first morning urines brought to your office with concentrations between 400 and 700 mOsm/kg H_2O. Diagnoses to be considered in her subsequent evaluation include

(1) chronic renal failure
(2) compulsive water drinking
(3) sickle cell disease
(4) nephrogenic diabetes insipidus (NDI)

SUMMARY OF DIRECTIONS

A	B	C	D	E
1,2,3	1,3	2,4	4	All are
only	only	only	only	correct

291. A 6-year-old girl is brought to the emergency room because her urine is red. Examination with a dipstick for heme is negative. Possible causes of the red color of the girl's urine include

(1) ingestion of blackberries
(2) ingestion of beets
(3) phenolphthalein catharsis
(4) presence of myoglobin

292. Hemolytic uremic syndrome can be described by which of the following statements?

(1) It commonly is preceded by infection
(2) It is characterized by development of acute renal failure
(3) Children 5 years of age or less are most often affected
(4) Blacks are affected more often than whites

293. A 14-year-old boy who has renal dysplasia develops a urinary tract infection. His serum creatinine is reported to be 6.2 mg per 100 ml. Which of the following antibiotics, as possible treatment for the boy's infection, would require dosage alteration in this situation?

(1) Ampicillin
(2) Amoxicillin
(3) Gentamicin
(4) Clindamycin

294. Abdominal ultrasound is a useful diagnostic tool that is able to

(1) localize kidneys for renal biopsy
(2) determine whether or not a renal mass is cystic
(3) differentiate multicystic kidney from hydronephrosis
(4) differentiate hydronephrosis from urinomas, hematomas, or lymphoceles

295. Congenital nephrosis is characterized by

(1) circulating immune complexes
(2) frequent gross hematuria
(3) responsiveness to steroid therapy
(4) an increased incidence within families

DIRECTIONS: Each group of questions below consists of lettered headings followed by a set of numbered items. For each numbered item select the **one** lettered heading with which it is **most** closely associated. Each lettered heading may be used **once, more than once, or not at all.**

Questions 296–300

For each condition listed below, match the category to which it belongs.

(A) Primary renal tubular defect
(B) Developmental structural abnormality
(C) Metabolic disorder leading to renal damage
(D) Multisystem disorder
(E) Primary renal disease with multiple renal manifestations
(F) No renal involvement

296. Cystinuria   A

297. Wilson's disease   C

298. Alport's syndrome   E

299. Prune belly syndrome   D

300. Crossed, fused ectopia   B

Questions 301–305

For each diagnosis that follows, select the mode of inheritance with which it is usually associated.

(A) Autosomal dominant
(B) Autosomal recessive
(C) X-linked dominant
(D) X-linked recessive
(E) None of the above

C 301. Hypophosphatemic rickets

B 302. Childhood-type polycystic kidneys

E 303. Systemic lupus erythematosus

B 304. Cystinosis

A 305. Adult-type polycystic kidneys

DIRECTIONS: The group of questions below consists of four lettered headings followed by a set of numbered items. For each numbered item select

A	if the item is associated with	(A) **only**
B	if the item is associated with	(B) **only**
C	if the item is associated with	**both** (A) and (B)
D	if the item is associated with	**neither** (A) nor (B)

Each lettered heading may be used **once, more than once, or not at all.**

Questions 306–311

(A) Nephrotic syndrome
(B) Acute glomerulonephritis
(C) Both
(D) Neither

306. Serum albumin concentration of 1.9 g/L

307. Edema

308. Need to carefully monitor and restrict water intake

309. Cured by diuretics

310. Hypovolemia

311. Commonly accompanied by hypertension

The Urinary Tract
Answers

268. The answer is C. *(Behrman, ed 12. p 1382.)* Drug-related nephrotic syndrome has been described in connection with the use of trimethadione, penicillamine, tolbutamide, and certain heavy metals. A variety of allergic causes, including Hymenoptera stings, pollens, insect bites, and snakebites, also have been implicated as etiologic agents. Nephrosis can develop in conjunction with malignancy and diseases such as amyloidosis.

269. The answer is D. *(Behrman, ed 12. pp 1369–1370. Rudolph, ed 17. p 1209.)* No bacteria at all should grow in a properly obtained urine sample from a suprapubic tap or from retrograde catheterization of the upper urinary tract unless infection is present. Any bacterial growth at all from a properly obtained suprapubic tap is significant. First-morning urine usually is concentrated, and a higher colony count is expected. Ileal-loop bags are usually contaminated. Bladder catheterization of a normal person may produce urine that shows bacterial contamination of the specimen.

270. The answer is C. *(Behrman, ed 12. pp 1328–1329.)* Membranoproliferative glomerulonephritis, a chronic, diffuse, proliferative nephritis, occurs in two main forms that are indistinguishable histologically. The micrograph shown in the question depicts type I membranoproliferative glomerulonephritis (MPGN type I) with interposition of mesangial matrix between the basement membrane and the endothelial layer. Subendothelial deposits are also seen. Type I MPGN is more common than type II, which is called "dense deposit disease" because dense-appearing deposits occur within the basement membrane. Complement abnormalities are usually found in both MPGN type I and type II. In type I C3 is variably decreased and depression of C1q and C4 is often seen. In type II C3 is said to be more persistently decreased, suggesting alternative pathway activation. Progressive renal failure may occur in either form.

271. The answer is C. *(Behrman, ed 12. pp 1311, 1323, 1347, 1355, 1372.)* In individuals affected by childhood nephrosis, there is a reduced ability to excrete a free water load; thus, urine is highly concentrated. Sickle-cell patients have isothenuria, probably caused by the sickling of erythrocytes in the vasa recta. Patients who have diabetes insipidus cannot concentrate their urine, either because of a lack of vasopressin (central diabetes insipidus) or an unresponsiveness to vasopressin (nephrogenic diabetes insipidus). Patients who have pyelonephritis may not be able to concentrate urine.

272. The answer is D. *(Behrman, ed 12. pp 580, 1337, 1372–1373, 1382–1383.)* In Potter's syndrome, the kidneys are absent; consequently, pyuria cannot be present. Potter's syndrome is a lethal abnormality that may be suspected at birth by the presence of oligohydramnios, a wizened appearance, and a characteristic wide semicircular fold of skin that extends downward and laterally from the inner canthus of both eyes. There may also be pulmonary hypoplasia. Sterile pyuria, as evidenced by the depicted white blood cells, may occur in febrile illness dehydration, acute nephritides, renal cystic disease, toxic nephropathy, and renal transplant rejection, as well as in the other disorders listed in the question.

273. The answer is A. *(Behrman, ed 12. p 1101.)* Average blood pressure tends to increase with age. Thus, a value of 120/80 mm Hg, clearly acceptable for most children, is in the hypertensive range for children in the first few years of life. In the newborn period, a systolic pressure above 90 mm Hg is considered hypertensive.

274. The answer is C. *(Behrman, ed 12. pp 1303–1304, 1312–1313.)* If an exogenous substance is capable of being metabolized, bound by plasma proteins, or secreted or reabsorbed by the renal tubule, it will not measure glomerular function adequately. With current radiologic techniques, it is possible to perform glomerular filtration-rate studies with isotopes such as ^{51}CR-ethylenediaminotetraacetate (^{51}Cr-EDTA) or ^{125}I-iothalamate. Nonradiolabeled substances such as inulin, cyanocobalamin, and mannitol may also be used.

275. The answer is E. *(Behrman, ed 12. pp 1323–1324, 1332.)* Physical findings of individuals who have nephrosis usually stem from edema, which may progress to generalized edema (anasarca). The edema is typically pitting and shifts with position. Although edema may occur in association with acute nephritis, it usually is less marked than in nephrosis. The large abdomens of patients who have polycystic kidney disease are not edematous. Cystinosis and diabetes insipidus do not cause edema.

276. The answer is C. *(Behrman, ed 12. pp 1401–1402.)* Because it is an abdominal organ in children, the bladder, especially when full, is often ruptured by blunt trauma and lower abdominal wounds. Though small bladder tears may be treated conservatively by catheter drainage, surgical exploration is likely to be needed. Extensive urethral injuries may require surgical drainage of periurethral hematoma, primary surgical repair, or even urinary diversion procedures. Most ureteral injuries require prompt surgical intervention, though such injuries are rare because of the protected position of the ureter. A retrograde cystourethrogram and intravenous urography may be helpful, especially with pelvic fracture or suspected renal trauma.

277. The answer is E. *(Behrman, ed 12. p 1324.)* The patient described is of the sex and age most typical for minimal-change nephrotic syndrome, which accounts for about 80 percent of all cases of idiopathic nephrotic syndrome of childhood. The presence of highly selective proteinuria, normal renal function, a normal urinary sediment, and normal blood pressure would further increase the likelihood of minimal-change disease. Histologically, the glomeruli of children affected by minimal-change nephrotic diseases are normal, except for smudging of epithelial foot processes on electron microscopy.

278. The answer is C. *(Behrman, ed 12. pp 1195–1200.)* Important clinical signs of hypertension in children may include headache, dizziness, visual disturbances, irritability, and nocturnal wakening. Hypertensive encephalopathy may be preceded or accompanied by vomiting, hyperreflexia, ataxia, and focal or generalized seizures. Facial palsy may be the sole manifestation of severe hypertension. When marked fundal changes are present or when there are signs of vascular compromise, emergency treatment of the accompanying hypertension is warranted. Such hypertensive individuals require immediate hospitalization for diagnosis and therapy.

279. The answer is D. *(Behrman, ed 12. pp 228–249.)* Owing to relatively good preservation of circulatory volume, patients who have hypertonic (hypernatremic) dehydration may look stable clinically. However, because the central nervous system is especially liable to insult, therapy must be approached cautiously. Brain edema, for example, can result from the too rapid administration of dilute solution. Careful and gradual replacement therapy is needed in most cases.

280. The answer is D. *(Behrman, ed 12. pp 1327–1328, 1330, 1332, 1335, 1336–1338.)* The figure accompanying the question depicts a red blood cell cast characteristically found in the urine of patients with glomerular disease. Important exceptions include the minimal lesion form of the nephrotic syndrome and membranous glomerulopathy. In these, the urine contains large amounts of protein and hyaline casts but few red blood cells.

281. The answer is B. *(Behrman, ed 12. pp 1307–1308.)* The kidneys of a newborn infant already contain their full complement of nephrons. Glomerular filtration rate and renal plasma flow steadily increase to close to normal adult values (corrected for surface area) by the end of the first year of life. Infants have a relatively low rate of sodium reabsorption, which increases proportionally as body weight increases. The secretion of substances such as paraaminohippuric acid also increases during the first year of life.

282. The answer is B. *(Behrman, ed 12. pp 575–579, 581, 605–606, 1338–1340.)* The rash of anaphylactoid purpura most often involves extensor surfaces of the extremities; the face, soles, palms, and trunk are rarely affected. Both systemic lupus erythematosus and dermatomyositis often are accompanied by typical facial rashes (butterfly and heliotrope, respectively). Individuals who have polyarteritis usually do not present with a rash. The scarlatiniform rash characteristic of streptococcal infections generally does not coincide with the development of poststreptococcal nephritis; impetiginous lesions, however, may still be present.

283. The answer is A. *(AAP-CID, ed 2. pp 71–73.)* Ethylene glycol is the main ingredient of antifreeze and is a clear liquid with a bittersweet taste; it is metabolized to oxalic acid. Renal damage occurs from the precipitation of oxalic acid crystals in the kidney. Ethanol is used in the early treatment to saturate the hepatic alcohol dehydrogenase and thus prevent further metabolism of the ethylene glycol. The other products on the list are nontoxic.

284. The answer is D (4). *(Behrman, ed 12. pp 1353–1354, 1357, 1375, 1385.)* The radiograph that accompanies the question shows the splayed-out calyces and large kidneys typical of adult-type polycystic kidneys, which can first appear in childhood. Multicystic kidneys are often unilateral; bilateral involvement in a 12-year-old child would be unlikely to be associated with the level of renal function pictured in the angiogram. Individuals who have nephronophthisis usually have normal or small-sized kidneys. Megacalyx is a rare entity in which the calyces appear large and can be mistaken for cysts; however, the renal cortex is normal.

285. The answer is A (1, 2, 3). *(Behrman, ed 12. pp 1347–1349.)* Nephrogenic diabetes insipidus is a hereditary congenital disorder in which the urine is hypotonic and produced in large volumes because the kidneys fail to respond to antidiuretic hormone. Most North American patients thus involved are descendants of Ulster Scots who came to Nova Scotia in 1761 on the ship Hopewell. Males are primarily affected, apparently through an X-linked recessive mode, though there can be a variable expression in heterozygous females. The defect is unknown, but the disorder is felt to result from primary unresponsiveness of the distal tubule and collecting duct to vasopressin. Although the condition is present at birth, the diagnosis is often not made until several months later when excessive thirst, frequent voidings of large volumes of dilute urine, dehydration, and failure to thrive become obvious. Maintenance of adequate fluid intake and diet and use of saluretic drugs are the bases of therapy of this incurable disease.

286. The answer is A (1, 2, 3). *(Behrman, ed 12. p 1336.)* With infected ventriculoatrial (VA) shunts, as well as in subacute bacterial endocarditis and osteomyelitis, a proliferative glomerulonephritis may occur. Immune complex glomerulonephritis with IgG or IgM plus antigens of the bacteria has been postulated to be involved. Serum C3 is usually low. Typical presentation may include both nephrotic and nephritic features. Hematuria, proteinuria, and red blood cell casts are often seen in the urine. Urine culture is usually negative, whereas blood cultures are frequently positive. Azotemia and hypertension are uncommon.

287. The answer is B (1, 3). *(Behrman, ed 12. p 1363.)* Chronic renal failure (CRF) often has a gradual, even insidious, onset with vague complaints, including nausea, loss of appetite, fatigue, and headache. Decreased urinary concentrating ability is reflected by nocturia, polyuria, and polydipsia. Later in the course of CRF, declining urine volume may be seen. Growth failure may occur, and accompanying renal osteodystrophy may be reflected by bone or joint pain. Muscle cramps and paresthesias are common, but hypotonia is not.

288. The answer is E (all). *(Behrman, ed 12. pp 1331–1334.)* The most common form of acute glomerulonephritis involves the deposition of complement, immunoglobulin G, and properdin in glomeruli following a skin or throat infection with certain nephritogenic strains of group A beta-hemolytic streptococci. Hematuria often colors the urine dark, and decreased urinary output may result in circulatory congestion and volume overload, which can induce dyspnea, pulmonary edema, periorbital edema, tachycardia, and hepatomegaly. This can be avoided by fluid restriction. Acute hypertension is common and may be associated with headache, vomiting, and encephalopathy with seizures.

289. The answer is A (1, 2, 3). *(Behrman, ed 12. pp 1379–1380.)* Causes of renal artery stenosis include abnormalities of the renal vessel wall, external encroachment by tumor or cyst, and embolism. Revascularization by means of arterial repair, vascular grafts, and autotransplantation is essential if hypertension is severe. Renovascular hypertension has been reported in infants as well as in older children.

290. The answer is A (1, 2, 3). *(Behrman, ed 12. pp 1311–1348.)* Children over age 2 years should have a first morning urine with a concentration of about 1100 mOsm (usual range: 870 to 1300). A variety of disorders impair renal concentrating ability including interstitial diseases, such as acute interstitial nephritis, and medullary injury, such as that associated with hydronephrosis or sickle cell disease. NDI patients have decreased ability to concentrate their urine and would be unlikely to have urinary concentration greater than 150 mOsm/kg H_2O. With compulsive water drinking, not possible to control in an outpatient setting, a first morning urine may not be concentrated. Further testing should include other parameters of renal function and more specific tests of water and solute handling.

291. The answer is A (1, 2, 3). *(Behrman, ed 12. pp 1307–1308.)* A number of pH-dependent substances can impart a red color to urine. Use of phenolphthalein, a cathartic agent, or phenindione, an anticoagulant, can cause red urine; ingestion of blackberries or beets also may lead to red coloration ("beeturia"). Because myoglobin tests heme-positive in a dipstick examination, myoglobinuria could not be the source of the red color of the urine of the girl described. Hematuria should be confirmed by dipstick testing as well as by microscopic examination of urinary sediment.

292. The answer is A (1, 2, 3). *(Behrman, ed 12. pp 1340–1343.)* Hemolytic uremic syndrome typically affects young children 5 years of age or less. The hallmarks of this disease, which often follows a viral-like gastrointestinal or upper respiratory tract illness, are severe hemolytic anemia, intravascular hemolysis, and platelet consumption that accompany acute renal failure. Hypertension, encephalopathy, and anuria also may occur. The syndrome seems to occur more frequently in whites than blacks.

293. The answer is A (1, 2, 3). *(Behrman, ed 12. p 1366.)* Many antibiotics require dosage alteration when administered to patients in renal failure. Major modification is required for gentamicin and other aminoglycosides. Penicillins, including ampicillin and amoxicillin, also require dosage modification. No dosage modification is needed with clindamycin therapy.

294. The answer is E (all). *(Behrman, ed 12. pp 1314, 1318.)* Renal ultrasound is noninvasive, and there is no unnecessary radiation exposure. Repeated studies are easily obtained for follow-up of problems. It is helpful in evaluating abdominal masses, especially in the newborn, and in examining transplanted kidneys. For example, renal ultrasound may be helpful in differentiating neoplasms from multicystic kidneys and hydronephrosis.

295. The answer is D (4). *(Behrman, ed 12. p 1329.)* Congenital nephrosis (infantile nephrosis), which occurs with an increased incidence in families having a history of the disease, is almost totally insensitive to any form of therapy. The characteristic lesion is cystic dilatation of the proximal tubules. Screening for elevated alpha-fetoprotein in amniotic fluid may be done in at-risk pregnancies.

296–300. The answers are: 296-A, 297-C, 298-E, 299-D, 300-B. *(Behrman, ed 12. pp 978, 1349–1352, 1375, 1391–1392.)* All the conditions listed have some familial associations, although prune belly syndrome (triad syndrome) and crossed, fused ectopia also occur sporadically. Patients with cystinuria have a defect of amino acid transport in both renal tubules and the gastrointestinal tract that leads to renal calculi from cystine. Treatment consists of maintaining high urinary flow rate and alkalinizing the urine, both of which decrease stone formation. D-Penicillamine may be effective in dissolving stones, as it forms a mixed disulfide of cysteine-penicillamine that is fifty times more soluble than cystine.

Patients with Wilson's disease may have copper deposition in the renal tubules, which may lead to renal tubular acidosis as well as hematuria, glycosuria, aminoaciduria, and hypercalcemia.

In Alport's syndrome, the most common inheritable renal disease, glomerular and tubular lesions both occur. Mean age of renal disease onset is 6 years, and end-stage renal disease occurs in half of males before age 30. Women are not usually so severely affected and may have only mild urinary abnormalities. Deafness and ocular abnormalities occur in some kindreds.

Prune belly syndrome, which consists of the triad of absent abdominal musculature, cryptorchidism, and dysplasia of the urinary tract, often with megacystis-megaureter, usually presents in infancy. The severity of renal involvement varies, with some patients developing chronic renal insufficiency.

Crossed, fused renal ectopia is generally not associated with clinical problems. However, the ectopic kidney may be more prone than a normally placed kidney to infection. If the ectopic kidney has an ectopic ureter, there may be constant perineal wetness.

301–305. The answers are: 301-C, 302-B, 303-E, 304-B, 305-A. *(Behrman, ed 12. pp 430, 575–577, 1336–1338, 1356–1357, 1656, 1660.)* All the disorders listed in the question are familial, even systemic lupus erythematosus, which appears to result from a combination of environmental and genetic causes. Lupus may result from a viral infection in genetically predisposed individuals.

Hypophosphatemic rickets (vitamin D–resistant rickets) is usually inherited as an X-linked dominant trait. Affected males therefore have a more severe form of this disease than affected females. It also seems to be transmitted on occasion as an autosomal recessive and even as an autosomal dominant trait.

Infantile polycystic kidney disease is an autosomal recessive disorder that is also associated with hepatic fibrosis developing as children get older. Renal failure may occur early in infancy but is of variable severity. It may lead to the need for dialysis and renal transplant. Liver disease, the main source of later problems, can lead to portal hypertension.

Adult-type polycystic kidney disease, inherited in an autosomal dominant fashion, is often seen in successive generations of the same family. If adult-type polycystic kidney disease is discovered, the family requires investigation.

Cystinosis is an autosomal recessive disease in which affected patients may develop renal failure in childhood or adolescence, or a more benign form in which renal failure does not occur. Now that some individuals who have cystine storage disease are receiving renal allografts, the pathologic effects of cystine storage in tissues other than the kidney may become clinically important.

306–311. The answers are: 306-A, 307-C, 308-B, 309-D, 310-A, 311-B. *(Finberg, pp 163–166.)* In the nephrotic syndrome albumin is lost in the urine and despite increased hepatic synthesis, serum levels drop. When the level drops low enough the oncotic pressure of the plasma becomes too low to balance the hydrostatic pressure. Plasma volume therefore decreases as edema occurs. Endocrine and renal mechanisms then partially compensate by retaining water and salt. Careful monitoring and restriction of water and salt intake is not usually required. With acute glomerulonephritis, on the other hand, oliguria frequently occurs as a direct consequence of the disease process itself and on occasion it can be profound with virtual anuria for several days. During this period of time it is vital to monitor and restrict fluid intake lest massive edema, hypervolemia, and even pulmonary edema and death occur. Hypertension commonly accompanies glomerulonephritis but only occasionally is associated with nephrotic syndrome.

Diuretics are sometimes used in both nephrotic syndrome and glomerulonephritis with temporary effect but are not curative. A combination of albumin infusions followed by a diuretic has been also used to temporarily decrease the edema in patients with nephrotic syndrome. Since both illnesses are usually self-limited, temporary measures are important.

The Neuromuscular System

DIRECTIONS: Each question below contains five suggested responses. Select the **one best** response to each question.

312. A diagnosis of Tourette's syndrome is based on the patient's history of

(A) encephalitis
(B) drug addiction
(C) positive response to methylphenidate
(D) repetitive writhing movements of the extremities
(E) brief, stereotypic movements of face and limbs

313. The virus causing subacute sclerosing panencephalitis is presumed to be which of the following?

(A) Rubella
(B) Epstein-Barr
(C) Herpes simplex
(D) Herpes zoster
(E) Measles virus

314. The most frequent complication of congenital rubella is believed to be

(A) cataracts
(B) microcephaly
(C) patent ductus arteriosus
(D) deafness
(E) thrombocytopenia

315. Which of the following aminoacidopathies is associated with acute infantile hemiplegia?

(A) Phenylketonuria
(B) Homocystinuria
(C) Cystathioninuria
(D) Maple syrup urine disease
(E) Histidinemia

316. The absence of hexosaminidase A activity in white blood cells confirms the diagnosis of which of the following lipidoses?

(A) Niemann-Pick disease
(B) Infantile Gaucher's disease
(C) Tay-Sachs disease
(D) Krabbe's disease
(E) Fabry's disease

317. Following a closed head injury, late seizures develop in approximately what percentage of children?

(A) Less than 5 percent
(B) 10 percent
(C) 15 percent
(D) 20 percent
(E) Over 25 percent

318. In children, the most common type of tumor of the central nervous system is

(A) meningioma
—(B) glioma (Astrocytoma)
(C) craniopharyngioma
(D) chordoma
(E) neurinoma

319. A subdural effusion most commonly accompanies meningitis caused by

(A) *Escherichia coli*
—(B) *Haemophilus influenzae*
(C) *Neisseria meningitidis*
(D) *Pseudomonas aeruginosa*
(E) *Streptococcus pneumoniae*

320. The pictured abnormality may be associated with

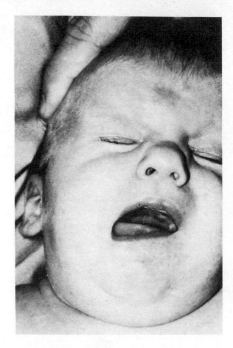

(A) loss of taste
— (B) cardiac and renal anomalies
(C) hyperacusis
(D) parotid tumor
(E) ptosis

321. A previously healthy 7-year-old child suddenly complains of a headache and falls to the floor. When examined in the emergency room, he is lethargic and has a left central facial weakness and left hemiparesis with conjugate ocular deviation to the right. The most likely diagnosis is

(A) hemiplegic migraine
(B) supratentorial tumor
(C) Todd's paralysis
(D) acute subdural hematoma
— (E) acute infantile hemiplegia

322. A 3-year-old child can be expected to do all the following EXCEPT

(A) undress
(B) copy a square
(C) alternate feet when climbing stairs
(D) name one color
(E) speak in short sentences

323. A 7-month-old infant develops head-nodding spells, which consist of a series of four to six nods a minute. These episodes are characteristic of which of the following disorders?

(A) Petit mal seizures
(B) Psychomotor seizures
(C) Focal motor seizures
(D) Infantile spasms
(E) Multiple tics

324. A 6-year-old child has a somewhat unsteady but nonspecific gait and is irritable. Physical examination reveals a very mild left facial weakness, brisk stretch reflexes in all four extremities, bilateral extensor plantar responses, and mild hypertonicity of the left upper and lower extremities; there is no muscular weakness. The most likely diagnosis is

(A) pontine glioma
(B) cerebellar astrocytoma
(C) right cerebral hemisphere tumor
(D) subacute sclerosing panencephalitis
(E) subacute necrotizing leuko-
    encephalopathy

325. Seizures associated with the pictured EEG segment present as

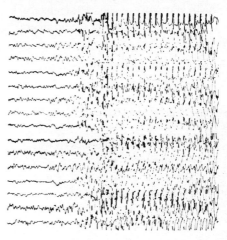

(A) petit mal
(B) grand mal
(C) psychomotor
(D) myoclonic
(E) spasmodic

326. A 10-year-old child complains of episodic abdominal discomfort; the child's mother says that these episodes are associated with periods of staring and followed by a brief period of lethargy. Which of the following disorders is most likely to be responsible for the child's symptoms?

(A) Psychomotor seizures
(B) Migraine
(C) Petit mal epilepsy
(D) Conversion reaction
(E) None of the above

327. Which of the following signs or symptoms must be present in a child's history in order to support the diagnosis of concussion following a head injury?

(A) Repeated vomiting
(B) Brief unconsciousness
(C) Drowsiness
(D) Seizure activity
(E) None of the above

328. A 10-year-old child who has acute lymphocytic leukemia is lethargic and unsteady. There is no evidence of hematuria or bleeding into the skin. Neurologic examination shows that the child has a mild spastic hemiparesis and hyperreflexia in all extremities; papilledema, however, is not present. Three months ago, the child was treated with 3000 rads of radiation to the head as well as with intrathecal methotrexate for meningeal leukemia.

The child's current neurologic disturbances most likely are the result of

(A) fungal infection
(B) hydrocephalus
(C) meningeal leukemia
(D) leukoencephalopathy
(E) intracerebral hemorrhage

329. Headache, vomiting, and papilledema are common symptoms and signs in children who have brain tumors. Which of the following signs also is frequently associated with craniopharyngioma?

(A) Sixth-nerve palsy
(B) Unilateral cerebellar ataxia
(C) Unilateral pupillary dilatation
(D) Unilateral anosmia
(E) Bitemporal hemianopia

330. The most common location in children for tumors of the nervous system is

(A) subtentorial
(B) supratentorial
(C) intraventricular
(D) in the spinal canal
(E) none of the above

331. Which of the following sets of clinical signs is most likely to be associated with the CAT scan (contrast positive) shown below?

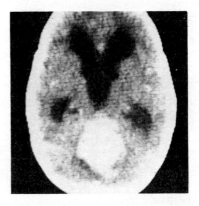

(A) Papilledema, hemiparesis, and ipsilateral sixth- and seventh-nerve palsies
(B) Papilledema, unilateral dysmetria, and falling to the same side
(C) Retinal angiomas, ataxia, and dysmetria
(D) Papilledema and ataxia without dysmetria
(E) None of the above

332. Erb's palsy is described best as

(A) weakness of a wrist and ipsilateral Horner's syndrome
(B) weakness of an arm from a fracture of the head of the humerus
—(C) weakness of an arm from a traction injury of the upper brachial plexus
(D) total ipsilateral arm weakness resulting from a fracture of a clavicle
(E) pseudoparalysis of an arm caused by syphilitic osteochondritis

333. A newborn infant has marked muscular weakness of the extremities and tongue fasciculations. The mother reports her child was relatively inactive in utero. The most likely diagnosis is

— (A) infantile spinal muscular atrophy
(B) Duchenne's muscular dystrophy
(C) myotonic dystrophy
(D) myasthenia gravis
(E) fiber type I disproportion

334. The calcific densities in the skull x-ray shown below are likely to have been caused by

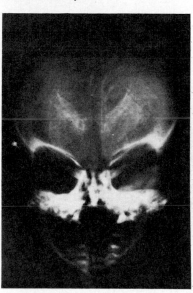

—(A) congenital cytomegalovirus infection
(B) congenital toxoplasmosis
(C) congenital syphilis
(D) tuberculous meningitis
(E) craniopharyngioma

335. An infant who has achromic skin patches develops infantile spasms. The disorder most likely to be affecting this infant is

(A) neurofibromatosis
— (B) tuberous sclerosis
(C) incontinentia pigmenti
(D) pityriasis rosea
(E) psoriasis

336. The patient whose CAT scan is pictured complained of recurrent headache and vomiting and had papilledema on examination of the fundi. Other features of her disease might include which one of the following?

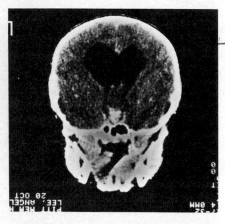

(A) History of a recent head injury
(B) Short stature
(C) Hyperthyroidism
(D) Achromic skin patches
(E) Multiple café au lait lesions

337. A 2-year-old patient with acute bacterial meningitis, diagnosed and treated earlier in the day, has developed oliguria. The most dangerous course of action is to

(A) do nothing
(B) increase the intravenous fluid rate by 20 percent for several hours
(C) give a renal challenge with an IV push over 10 minutes of 20 ml/kg of 5% dextrose in water
(D) decrease the IV fluid rate by 10 percent for several hours
(E) pass a catheter into the urinary bladder

DIRECTIONS: Each question below contains four suggested responses of which **one or more** is correct. Select

A	if	**1, 2, and 3**	are correct
B	if	**1 and 3**	are correct
C	if	**2 and 4**	are correct
D	if	**4**	is correct
E	if	**1, 2, 3, and 4**	are correct

338. Symmetrically small pupils in an unconscious patient may be found in

(1) metabolic coma
(2) pontine hemorrhage
(3) heroin-induced coma
(4) atropine-induced coma

339. Congenital defects frequently associated with the radiographic findings illustrated below include

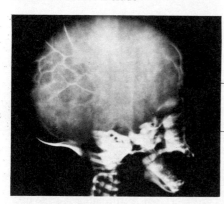

(1) meningomyelocele
(2) cleft lip and palate
(3) encephalocele
(4) craniosynostosis

340. Gowers' maneuver is used by children who have

(1) pseudohypertrophic muscular dystrophy
(2) limb-girdle dystrophy
(3) late-onset spinal muscular atrophy
(4) congenital myopathy

341. A 10-year-old child has pes cavus and scoliosis; other disorders likely to be exhibited by this child include

(1) diminished vibration and position sense
(2) gait and station ataxia
(3) nystagmus
(4) hyperreflexia

342. By 3 months of age most normal full-term infants can be expected to

(1) move their heads from side to side 180 degrees while following a moving object
(2) lift their heads from a prone position 45 degrees off the examining table
(3) smile when encouraged
(4) maintain a seated position

343. Frontal baldness, cataracts, distal muscle weakness, ptosis, and facial muscle weakness are some of the symptoms of myotonic dystrophy in adults. Children who have this disease commonly exhibit

(1) psychomotor retardation
(2) seizure activity
(3) respiratory distress
(4) clinical evidence of myotonia in early infancy

SUMMARY OF DIRECTIONS

A	B	C	D	E
1,2,3	1,3	2,4	4	All are
only	only	only	only	correct

344. Characteristics of childhood migraine include

(1) strong family history for migraine
(2) bifrontal headaches
(3) male preponderance before age 12 years
(4) duration of headaches more than 24 hours

345. Intracranial calcifications can appear in infants who have a congenital infection with

(1) *Treponema pallidum*
(2) *Toxoplasma gondii*
(3) rubella virus
(4) cytomegalovirus

346. Common sites of intracranial bleeding in full-term infants include

(1) intraventricular
(2) posterior fossa
(3) subarachnoid
(4) subdural

347. Examination of the cerebrospinal fluid of an 8-year-old, stuporous, mildly febrile child shows the following: white blood cells, 200/mm^3 (all lymphocytes); protein, 150 mg per 100 ml; and glucose, 15 mg per 100 ml. The differential diagnosis should include

(1) aseptic meningitis
(2) tuberculous meningitis
(3) meningeal leukemia
(4) medulloblastoma

348. Low cerebrospinal fluid (CSF) sugar is commonly associated with bacterial meningitis, but it may also be found in which of the following disorders?

(1) Hypoglycemia
(2) Subarachnoid hemorrhage
(3) Mumps meningitis
(4) Spinal cord tumor

349. Although valproic acid is widely used as an anticonvulsant, particularly for patients with petit mal seizures, there are side effects, which include

(1) hepatotoxicity
(2) hypotension
(3) interference with other anticonvulsants
(4) drug rash

350. The differential diagnosis for a newborn infant who has multiple joint contractures should include

(1) spinal muscular atrophy
(2) congenital muscular dystrophy
(3) congenital myopathies
(4) myelomeningocele

351. No precise definition exists for grand mal status epilepticus. This disorder generally can be defined by which of the following criteria?

(1) One seizure lasting no less than a half hour
(2) Continuous tonic-clonic activity for 1 hour
(3) Repeated seizures with no return to consciousness between them
(4) Several sets of repeated focal seizures occurring in a 24-hour period

352. The calcifications shown on the skull x-ray below can be associated with which of the following?

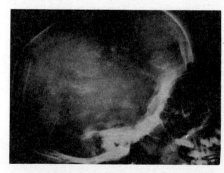

(1) Von Hippel–Lindau disease
(2) Ataxia-telangiectasia
(3) Tuberous sclerosis
(4) Sturge-Weber syndrome

353. A 6-year-old child is hospitalized for observation because of a short period of unconsciousness after a fall from a playground swing. Which of the following signs or symptoms would suggest the development of an extradural hematoma?

(1) Unilateral pupillary dilatation
(2) Focal seizures
(3) Recurrence of depressed consciousness
(4) Hemiplegia

354. Many diseases of the nervous system are inherited. Of the following, those that are considered to be autosomal dominant include

(1) familial dysautonomia A.R
(2) Huntington's chorea AD
(3) Wilson's disease A.R
(4) neurofibromatosis AD

355. The differential diagnosis of acute ataxia of childhood should include

(1) drug intoxication
(2) bacterial meningitis
(3) postinfectious viral syndrome
(4) neuroblastoma

356. A newborn infant is noted to have facial diplegia and difficulty sucking and swallowing. Which of the following disorders should be included in the differential diagnosis?

(1) Infantile spinal muscular atrophy
(2) Myasthenia gravis
(3) Myotonic dystrophy
(4) Duchenne's muscular dystrophy

2 _ 3 ans

SUMMARY OF DIRECTIONS

A	B	C	D	E
1,2,3	1,3	2,4	4	All are
only	only	only	only	correct

357. Bloody cerebrospinal fluid (CSF) produced by a traumatic lumbar puncture can be distinguished from true bloody CSF from other causes by which of the following methods?

(1) Counting red blood cells in more than one tube
(2) Looking for xanthochromia
(3) Repeating the lumbar puncture at a higher interspace
(4) Observing clotting in the CSF

358. A "cherry red spot" in the eye is a well-known finding in Tay-Sachs disease. It may also be found in children with

(1) GM1 type 1 generalized gangliosidosis
(2) GM2 type 2 Sandhoff's disease
(3) Niemann-Pick disease, type A
(4) metachromatic leukodystrophy

359. Neonatal seizures can develop as the result of

(1) hypocalcemia
(2) hypoxia
(3) birth trauma
(4) anomalies of the central nervous system

360. True statements about febrile seizures include which of the following?

(1) They usually occur in association with infection outside of the central nervous system
(2) Most last less than 15 minutes
(3) Affected children usually are between 6 months and 3 years of age
(4) Generalized tonic-clonic activity is typical

361. Which of the following can be associated with jitteriness in the newborn?

(1) Hypoxic encephalopathy
(2) Hypoglycemia
(3) Drug withdrawal
(4) Hypocalcemia

362. Physical findings characteristic of children who have Sturge-Weber syndrome include

(1) hemiplegia
(2) a "port wine" nevus on the forehead
(3) angiomas of the lips and mouth
(4) an angioma of the retina

363. Laboratory findings consistently associated with Reye's syndrome include which of the following?

(1) Prolonged prothrombin time
(2) Elevated levels of serum transaminases
(3) Elevated blood ammonia levels
(4) Elevated blood glucose levels

hypoglycemia

364. An asymmetric Moro reflex can be elicited at least occasionally from infants who have

— (1) a fractured clavicle
— (2) infantile hemiplegia
— (3) a brachial plexus palsy
   (4) neonatal myasthenia gravis

365. A 4-year-old patient in coma with severe brain injury has developed diabetes insipidus with urine output of 100 ml per hour. This can be managed by

— (1) replacing excessive urine output with a solution of 5% glucose and 10 mEq/L of NaCl
— (2) giving vasopressin in oil intramuscularly
— (3) giving extra water via the nasogastric tube to replace the excessive urine
   (4) water restriction

The Neuromuscular System

Answers

312. The answer is E. *(Shapiro, Semin Neurol 2:375, 1982.)* The clinical characteristics of Tourette's syndrome are multiple tics involving the face, head and neck, shoulders, and limbs, and vocal tics, such as sniffing, snorting, and throat clearing. In contrast to other movement disorders, this disorder does not have a recognized antecedent illness or CNS insult as its cause. There may be a genetic factor, as epidemiologic studies have identified other family members with the same disorder. The drug of choice for treatment is haloperidol. Clonidine has been used as a second choice.

313. The answer is E. *(Bell, vol 12. p 293.)* The infective agent considered to cause subacute sclerosing panencephalitis is measles virus. The presumption is based on the associated central nervous system pathology, which is consistent with encephalitis and features intranuclear and intracytoplasmic inclusion bodies. In addition, measles (rubeola) antibody titers in serum and cerebrospinal fluid are higher than those found in children recovering from measles, a finding that suggests a continuing infective process.

314. The answer is D. *(Bell, vol 12. pp 272–273.)* Microcephaly, cataracts, congenital heart defects, vasomotor instability, and developmental retardation are among the many disturbances of the congenital rubella syndrome. Deafness, however, is thought to be the single most common defect associated with this disorder. Although the hearing loss seems to involve the inner ear and result primarily in a sensorineural defect, middle-ear damage also has been suggested as an etiologic factor.

315. The answer is B. *(Menkes, ed 2. pp 1–7, 14–16, 21–25.)* Homocystinuria can cause thromboembolic phenomena in the pulmonary and systemic arteries and therefore in the cerebral vasculature; vascular occlusive disease is, in turn, one of the many causes of acute infantile hemiplegia. None of the other disorders listed in the question are associated with acute hemiplegia. Phenylketonuria causes retardation and, on occasion, seizures; maple syrup urine disease, an abnormality of the metabolism of leucine, leads to seizures and rapid deterioration of the central nervous system in newborn infants; histidinemia seems to be associated with speech impairments and other minor neurologic difficulties; and cystathioninuria is most likely a benign aminoaciduria having no effect on the central nervous system.

316. The answer is C. *(Adams and Lyon, pp 43–46, 58–62, 272–274.)* Children who have Tay-Sachs disease are characterized by progressive developmental deterioration; physical signs include macular "cherry red" spots and exquisite sensitivity to noise. Diagnosis of this disorder can be confirmed biochemically by the absence of hexosaminidase A activity in white blood cells. Tay-Sachs disease is inherited as an autosomal recessive trait; about 80 percent of affected children are of Eastern European Jewish ancestry. The other disorders listed in the question are associated with enzyme deficiencies as follows: Niemann-Pick disease, sphingomyelinase; infantile Gaucher's disease, beta-glucosidase; Krabbe's disease (globoid cell leukodystrophy), galactocerebroside beta-galactosidase; and Fabry's disease, alpha-galactosidase.

317. The answer is A. *(Rudolph, ed 17. p 1650.)* Seizures resulting from head injury fall into two categories: The early type occurs within one week following the injury; the late type does not appear until 3 months to as much as 10 years later. Less than 5 percent of children with closed head injuries develop late seizures. Children, especially those under 5 years of age, are more likely to have early seizures than are adults, in whom later seizures are more common.

318. The answer is B. *(Rudolph, ed 17. pp 1622, 1627, 1630.)* Gliomas–for example, astrocytoma, pontine glioma, and optic glioma–constitute 75 percent of intracranial tumors in children and 45 percent in adults. After leukemia, intracranial tumors are the most common type of neoplastic disease among children. Only about 6 percent of brain tumors in children are metastatic from other sites.

319. The answer is B. *(Menkes, ed 2. pp 281–282.)* Although subdural effusions can follow all types of acute bacterial meningitis, they most commonly complicate meningitis caused by *Haemophilus influenzae*. How these effusions develop remains uncertain. Abnormal transillumination of the skull as well as certain clinical findings, such as progressive increase in head circumference or occurrence of focal neurologic signs, can suggest the presence of a subdural effusion.

320. The answer is B. *(Monreal, Pediatrics 65:146–149, 1980. Nelson, J Pediatr 81:16–20, 1972. Pape, J Pediatr 81:21–30, 1972.)* The pictured infant has the so-called asymmetric crying face and not a facial nerve palsy. The former has normal furrowing of the ipsilateral forehead, eye closure, and a normal appearing nasolabial fold during crying. The abnormality results from hypoplasia of the triangularis muscle, the muscle that pulls the corner of the mouth downward and outward. Palpation of the involved side of the lip will reveal diminished bulk compared with the uninvolved side. This anomaly has been associated with others involving the cardiovascular, musculoskeletal, and genitourinary systems.

321. The answer is E. *(Isler, pp 74–102. Menkes, ed 2. pp 264–267.)* The abrupt onset of a hemisyndrome, especially with the eyes looking away from the paralyzed side, strongly indicates a diagnosis of acute infantile hemiplegia. Most frequently this represents a thromboembolic occlusion of the middle cerebral artery or one of its major branches. Hemiplegic migraine commonly occurs in children with a history of migraine headaches. Todd's paralysis follows after a focal or jacksonian seizure and generally does not last more than 24 to 48 hours. The eyes usually look toward the paralyzed side. The clinical onset of a supratentorial brain tumor is subacute with repeated headaches and gradually developing weakness. A history of trauma usually precedes the signs of an acute subdural hematoma. Clinical signs may appear fairly rapidly, but not with the abruptness of occlusive vascular disease.

322. The answer is B. *(Illingworth, ed 7. pp 135, 137, 143, 145, 161.)* By 3 years of age children become quite skilled in many areas. Most can say many words and speak in sentences. They are usually toilet trained and can dress and undress themselves with the exception of shoelaces and sometimes buttons. Although they can alternate feet when climbing stairs, they still place both feet on each step when going down stairs. They can identify at least one color by name but have not progressed beyond copying a circle and a crude cross. Only at 4 to 5 years of age can a child copy a square.

323. The answer is D. *(Hrachovy, J Pediatr 103:641–645, 1983. Menkes, ed 2. pp 558–560. Singer, J Pediatr 96:485–489, 1980.)* The onset of infantile spasms most commonly occurs in children between the ages of 3 and 8 months. The seizures, which occur in clusters, may take the form of head nodding (with or without arm extension) or spasms of more severe flexion ("salaam seizure"). ACTH (adrenocorticotropin) has been significantly effective in controlling these seizures, though prednisone therapy is thought by some to be equally therapeutic. Normal intellectual development in any infant who has developed infantile spasms is unlikely if there is evidence of prenatal or perinatal neurologic insults, metabolic disorders, or structural abnormalities of the brain. Petit mal seizures, psychomotor seizures, and multiple tics do not occur in infants of this age group. Focal motor seizures may occur at any age but usually involve limbs or facial muscles.

324. The answer is A. *(Altman, pp 314–315.)* A child who has a subacute disorder of the central nervous system producing cranial-nerve abnormalities (especially of the seventh nerve and the lower bulbar nerves), long-tract signs, unsteady gait secondary to spasticity, and some behavioral changes is most likely to have a pontine glioma. Tumors of the cerebellar hemispheres may in later stages produce long-tract signs, but the gait disturbance would be ataxia. Dysmetria and nystagmus also would be present. Supratentorial tumors are quite uncommon in 6-year-old children; headache and vomiting would be likely presenting symptoms and papilledema a finding on physical examination.

325. The answer is A. *(Sato, Neurology 32:157–163, 1982.)* The pictured EEG is fairly typical of petit mal absence: generalized 3 c/s spike and slow wave activity. The spells are usually brief, consisting of staring with eye blinking, lack of awareness, and minor motor activity such as chewing or lip smacking.

326. The answer is A. *(Menkes, ed 2. pp 553–556.)* The consecutive appearances of abdominal distress, staring, and sleepiness or lethargy strongly indicate a paroxysmal disorder. Children who have psychomotor seizures often present in this manner. Other symptoms that have been described include stereotyped motor activity (such as buttoning and unbuttoning of clothes), a sensation of unexplained fearfulness, and déjà vu. Affected children may have a history of febrile seizures.

327. The answer is B. *(Behrman, ed 12. p 1594.)* Although vomiting and lethargy frequently are associated with a closed head injury, a brief period of unconsciousness following the injury defines a concussion. Children old enough to relate their own histories may give evidence of amnesia concerning the events preceding their head injuries (retrograde amnesia) and following their injuries (antegrade amnesia); these historical findings will confirm the diagnosis of concussion. The severity of the injury is generally directly related to the length of time the child was unconscious and the extent of the retrograde amnesia.

328. The answer is D. *(Neville, Develop Med Child Neurol 14:75–78, 1972. Price, Cancer 35:306–318, 1975. Rubenstein, Cancer 35:291–305, 1975.)* Acute leukemia in children is associated with a number of complications involving the central nervous system. The child described in the question most likely has necrotizing leukoencephalopathy, a recently recognized complication of combined irradiation and intrathecal methotrexate therapy. It has been suggested that irradiation in excess of 2500 rads permits methotrexate to pass into the white matter, resulting in progressive necrosis. Meningeal leukemia, which has become more common with the advent of improved chemotherapy, can lead to hydrocephalus, presumably by infiltration of the arachnoid membrane and consequent obstruction of the flow and absorption of cerebrospinal fluid. Intracerebral hemorrhages usually occur from thrombocytopenia and produce evidence of bleeding into the skin and other organs. Because of immunosuppression, leukemic children are also prone to infection by fungi and yeast.

329. The answer is E. *(Swaiman, ed 2. p 644.)* Upward growth of a craniopharyngioma results in compression of the optic chiasm. Particularly affected are the fibers derived from the nasal portions of both retinas (in other words, from those parts of the eyes receiving stimulation from the temporal visual field). Early in the growth of a craniopharyngioma a unilateral superior quadrantanopic defect can develop; and an irregularly growing tumor can impinge upon the optic chiasm and cause homonymous hemianopia.

330. The answer is A. *(Menkes, ed 2. p 498.)* Between 60 and 70 percent of intracranial tumors in children are located below the tentorium. Of these tumors, the two most common types are medulloblastoma and cerebellar astrocytoma. In adults and infants, most intracranial tumors originate above the tentorium; only 25 to 30 percent of brain tumors in adults are subtentorial.

331. The answer is D. *(Behrman, ed 12. pp 1586–1587.)* The CAT scan presented in the question shows dilation of the lateral and third ventricles and a mass filling the fourth ventricle. These findings point to a midline, fourth ventricular tumor, such as a medulloblastoma or ependymoma; clinical signs of these tumors include papilledema and ataxia without dysmetria. The clinical signs of lateralized dysmetria and falling to the same side usually are associated with hemispheric cystic cerebellar astrocytoma; a CAT scan of patients with this disorder can be expected to show a lateralized cystic mass displacing the fourth ventricle to one side. A pontine glioma should be suspected in children who have long-tract signs, either unilaterally or bilaterally, and cranial nerve palsies, especially of the third, sixth, and seventh nerves. Cerebellar hemangioma-blastoma usually occurs in association with a retinal angioma (von Hippel–Lindau syndrome). The clinical signs stemming from bleeding within the tumor depend on the location of the tumor in the cerebellum. Blood can be seen on a CAT scan **without** the use of a contrast agent.

332. The answer is C. *(Menkes, ed 2. pp 269–270.)* Erb's palsy can be caused by traction on an arm during a breech delivery or on the neck during a vertex delivery resulting in injury to the upper brachial plexus and causing weakness of the deltoid, biceps, brachialis, and wrist and finger extensor muscles. Recovery is dependent on the degree of nerve injury. Pain caused by osteochondritis of the humerus in an infant who has congenital syphilis (Parrot's pseudoparalysis) inhibits arm movement.

333. The answer is A. *(Behrman, ed 12. pp 1602–1603.)* Infantile spinal muscular atrophy (Werdnig-Hoffmann disease) is a progressive degenerative disease of anterior horn cells and bulbar motor nuclei. Fasciculations of the tongue can occur in affected infants; however, because tongue fasciculations can accompany crying in normal infants, only the demonstration of fasciculations while a child is at rest will support a diagnosis of infantile spinal muscular atrophy. Some mothers of affected neonates give a history of slowed or arrested fetal movement prior to the onset of labor. Because this disease has an autosomal recessive inheritance pattern, muscle biopsy and examination of histochemically stained specimens should be done to confirm the diagnosis.

334. The answer is A. *(Behrman, ed 12. pp 1565–1566.)* Periventricular calcifications are a characteristic finding in infants who have congenital cytomegalovirus infection. The encephalitic process especially affects the subependymal tissue around the lateral ventricles and thus results in the periventricular deposition of calcium.

Calcified tuberculomas, if visible radiographically, are not periventricular. Granulomatous encephalitis caused by congenital toxoplasmosis is associated with scattered and soft-appearing intracranial calcification, and suprasellar calcifications are typical of craniopharyngiomas. Congenital syphilis does not produce intracranial calcifications.

335. The answer is B. *(Behrman, ed 12. p 1678. Westmoreland, pp 55–57.)* In infants, achromic skin patches, especially in association with infantile spasms, are characteristic of tuberous sclerosis. Other dermal abnormalities (adenoma sebaceum and subungual fibromata) associated with this disorder appear later in childhood. Although children who have neurofibromatosis may have a few achromic patches, the identifying dermal lesions are café au lait spots. Incontinentia pigmenti also is associated with seizures; the skin lesions typical of this disorder begin as bullous eruptions that later become hyperpigmented lesions. Pityriasis rosea and psoriasis are not associated with infantile spasms.

336. The answer is B. *(Thomsett, J Pediatr 97:728–735, 1980.)* This CAT scan of a patient with craniopharyngioma shows hydrocephalus involving the lateral ventricles, a calcific density within the sella, and a mass extending from it compromising the third ventricle. In a recent study of 42 children with craniopharyngioma 43 percent had headache and 35 percent had visual complaints as their initial complaint. Only three were referred for evaluation of delayed growth. However, about one third of the children were more than two standard deviations below height for their age. Almost all the children had endocrinologic disturbances of the hypothalamic pituitary axis prior to surgery. Plain skull films can show abnormalities of the sella and calcification within or above the sella.

337. The answer is C. *(Finberg, p 169.)* The most dangerous action in a patient with acute bacterial meningitis or other central nervous system diseases predisposing to brain swelling is to give a rapid intravenous push of a solution with a low effective osmolality. This can cause a rapid shift of water into the brain with brain swelling and the potential for brain damage and death. The other actions listed are all less dangerous, but doing nothing at this stage is probably the best course.

338. The answer is A (1, 2, 3). *(Plum, ed 3. pp 46–47.)* Pinpoint pupils are found in coma from heroin and pontine hemorrhage. The light reflex is preserved in the former, though it may be difficult to confirm. Small light-reactive pupils are found in metabolic coma, whereas a midbrain injury would produce small, but unresponsive, pupils. Atropine produces dilated pupils, facial flushing, delirium, or stupor.

339. The answer is B (1, 3). *(McRae, Acta Radiol 5:55, 1966.)* Lacunar skull results from abnormal membranous bone formation; it probably begins in utero and resolves by 6 months of age. The cause is not known but, contrary to popular belief, does not have any relation to increased intracranial pressure, even though it is associated frequently with encephalocele or meningomyelocele. Thinning of bone, which occurs in the thickest parts of the frontal, parietal, and upper portion of the occipital bones, creates the impression that there are holes in the skull.

340. The answer is E (all). *(Dubowitz, pp 24–26. Kelley, p 7.)* Gowers' maneuver is characteristic of individuals who have proximal muscle weakness of the pelvic girdle, regardless of the etiology. These individuals, when wishing to arise after lying down, must become prone and gradually stand by using their hands to "walk" up their legs. Not specific just for Duchenne's (pseudohypertrophic) muscular dystrophy, Gowers' maneuver also is used by children who have limb-girdle dystrophy, late-onset spinal muscular dystrophy, and congenital myopathy.

341. The answer is A (1, 2, 3). *(Menkes, ed 2. pp 118–122.)* Friedreich's ataxia, a spinocerebellar degenerative disease, is characterized by both cerebellar and posterior column dysfunction. Pes cavus (high arch) and scoliosis are skeletal hallmarks of this disorder, which can be inherited as either an autosomal dominant or an autosomal recessive trait. Neurologic symptoms frequently encountered include abnormal speech, diminished position and vibration sense, nystagmus, hyporeflexia, and gait and station ataxia. There is no curative treatment for children who have Friedreich's ataxia.

342. The answer is A (1, 2, 3). *(Behrman, ed 12. pp 36–38.)* Infants who are developing normally should be able to smile when smiled at or talked to by 8 weeks of age. By 3 months of age, infants should be able to follow a moving toy not only from side to side but also in the vertical plane. When placed on their abdomens, normal 3-month-old infants can raise their faces 45 to 90 degrees from the horizontal. Not until 6 to 8 months of age should infants be able to maintain a seated position.

343. The answer is B (1, 3). *(Rudolph, ed 17. p 1697.)* Psychomotor retardation may be the presenting complaint of children who have myotonic dystrophy. Ptosis, facial immobility, and neonatal respiratory distress are major features of this disorder in the newborn period. Not infrequently the mother may have the disease in a mild form, and a careful family history and examination of the parents, particularly the mother, may be necessary to elicit the diagnosis, particularly since clinical and electrical evidence of myotonia may not be present in an affected infant. Seizures are not prominent features of myotonic dystrophy.

344. The answer is A (1, 2, 3). *(Brown, Develop Med Child Neurol 19:683–692, 1977. Prensky, Neurology 29:506–510, 1979.)* In contrast to adults, children with migraine most often have "common" migraine: bifrontal headache without an aura or diffuse throbbing headache of only a few hours' duration. As with adults, the headaches may be terminated with vomiting or sleep. Migraine may begin as early as 2 to 3 years of age, with boys being affected somewhat more than girls until preteen or early teen years when girls, like adult young women, are more likely to have migraine.

345. The answer is C (2, 4). *(Menkes, ed 2. pp 307, 309.)* Neonates who have congenital syphilis, rubella, toxoplasmosis, or cytomegalic inclusion disease all have jaundice and hepatosplenomegaly. Only the last two, however, are associated with intracranial calcification. In infants who have congenital toxoplasmosis, intracranial calcifications occur in scattered locations in the brain. Calcium deposits in infants who have a cytomegaloviral infection, on the other hand, appear in subependymal tissue; as a consequence, these calcifications tend to outline the ventricular system.

346. The answer is C (2, 4). *(Volpe, pp 762–769.)* Intraventricular or germinal matrix hemorrhage with rupture into the lateral ventricle is most commonly seen in hypoxic premature infants. Hypoxia and prematurity are also the common predisposing factors for subarachnoid hemorrhage. In contrast, subdural and posterior fossa hemorrhages are sequelae of difficult deliveries with torsion and tearing of major venous channels. Subdural hemorrhages result from rupture of superficial veins, and posterior fossa hemorrhages from tears of tentorial veins or veins of Galen.

347. The answer is E (all). *(Behrman, ed 12. p 618.)* Aseptic meningitis, tuberculous meningitis, meningeal leukemia, and medulloblastoma can cause pleocytosis as well as elevated protein and lowered glucose concentrations in cerebrospinal fluid. Of the four diseases, tuberculous meningitis is associated with the lowest cerebrospinal fluid glucose levels. The cellular response to viral (aseptic) meningitis will be predominantly lymphocytic. Cells found in the cerebrospinal fluid of a child who has meningeal leukemia most commonly are lymphocytes or lymphoblasts. Children who have a medulloblastoma generally present with the signs and symptoms caused by a mass in the posterior cranial fossa; their pleocytotic cerebrospinal fluid contains unusual-appearing cells of the monocytic variety. The decrease in the cerebrospinal glucose concentration associated with these disorders has been attributed to a disturbance of glucose transport as a result of meningeal irritation.

348. The answer is E (all). *(Fishman, pp 208–214.)* Low cerebrospinal fluid (CSF) sugar (hypoglycorrachia) may be found in all the conditions listed in the question. The amount of glucose in CSF reflects both entry and exit of the glucose in and out of the CSF space as well as its utilization by cellular elements. This may explain the low CSF glucose in subarachnoid hemorrhage, but it does not account for the low CSF sugar below the block caused by a malignant tumor, the cause of which remains unknown. The CSF sugar level tends to be 60 to 80 percent of that in the plasma, and therefore, hypoglycorrachia is found in conjunction with hypoglycemia.

349. The answer is B (1, 3). *(Browne, N Engl J Med 302:661–665, 1980.)* There have been several reported deaths caused by liver failure in patients being treated with valproic acid. It is necessary to measure a patient's serum aspartate aminotransferase (serum glutamic-oxaloacetic transaminase, SGOT) and alanine aminotransferase (serum glutamic-pyruvic transaminase, SGPT) on a monthly basis when introducing the drug, and at 3- to 6-month intervals when the maintenance dosage has been achieved. If elevation of these enzymes occurs, they may respond to reduction of dosage; however, if they exceed three times the upper limit of normal or are associated with other indications of altered liver function, the medication should be discontinued. While valproic acid may increase the serum level of phenobarbital and cause signs of toxicity, it also may decrease the total phenytoin level without increasing the free (active) serum phenytoin. This could result in increased seizure activity.

350. The answer is E (all). *(Dubowitz, pp 232–235. Walton, ed 4. pp 645–646.)* Multiple joint contractures in newborn infants are symptoms of diseases of muscle or of disturbances in muscle innervation. The clinical picture associated with these contractures has been called arthrogryposis multiplex congenita. Infants who have a myelomeningocele frequently have contractures of ankle and knee joints as a result of the spinal cord defect and immobilization of the lower extremities in utero.

351. The answer is A (1, 2, 3). *(Delgado-Escueta, pp 3–14.)* Although no exact definition of grand mal status epilepticus now exists, there is general agreement that the term implies either repeated seizures without a lucid, responsive interval or a grand mal seizure lasting at least a half hour. Some neurologists prefer to use the criterion of continuous tonic-clonic activity for 1 hour. Grand mal status epilepticus occurs more commonly than petit mal or psychomotor status and, if not treated, is the most serious and potentially lethal of the three. It can develop secondarily to a central nervous system infection, a toxic metabolic state, or a primary seizure disorder.

352. The answer is D (4). *(Behrman, ed 12. p 1575.)* The parallel linear calcifications ("tram line" calcifications) seen in the skull x-ray presented in the question are typical of Sturge-Weber syndrome. These calcifications lie within the cerebral cortex; they are not within the intracranial vascular malformations common in individuals who have this syndrome. Sturge-Weber syndrome is associated with a high incidence of mental retardation.

353. The answer is E (all). *(Menkes, ed 2. pp 421–424. Rudolph, ed 17. pp 1647–1648.)* Compression of the third cranial nerve and distortion of the brainstem, resulting in unilateral pupillary dilatation, hemiplegia, focal seizures, and depressed consciousness, suggest a progressively enlarging mass, most likely an extradural hematoma. Such a hematoma displaces the temporal lobe into the tentorial notch and presses on the ipsilateral third cranial nerve. Pupillary dilatation occurs before third cranial nerve pareses. Brainstem compression by this additional tissue mass leads to progressive deterioration in consciousness.

354. The answer is C (2, 4). *(Swaiman, ed 2. pp 336–339.)* Huntington's chorea and neurofibromatosis share only their inheritance pattern, that of an autosomal dominant disorder. Familial dysautonomia (Riley-Day syndrome) and Wilson's disease (hepatolenticular degeneration) are autosomal recessive diseases. It is important to be aware of the genetic nature of various neurologic disorders in order to provide accurate genetic counseling.

355. The answer is E (all). *(Rudolph, ed 17. pp 1708, 1773–1775.)* Cerebellar ataxia in childhood most commonly occurs in association with a mild viral syndrome or viral exanthem. Ingestion—whether intentional or accidental—of barbiturates, phenytoin, or alcohol also must be considered. Children who have bacterial meningitis can present, though rarely, with acute ataxia. Ataxia, opsoclonus (chaotic eye movements), and myoclonus constitute infantile polymyoclonia, which can occur in association with neuroblastoma.

356. The answer is A (1, 2, 3). *(Dubowitz, pp 139–142, 149, 192–193. Rudolph, ed 17. pp 1681–1683, 1689, 1697.)* Spinal muscular atrophy occurring in a neonate is associated with hypotonia and feeding difficulties; a muscle biopsy can confirm this diagnosis. Neonatal myasthenia gravis, though uncommon, must be considered in a newborn infant who has the symptoms described in the question. The symptoms presented also could represent myotonic dystrophy; this diagnosis is confirmed by examination of both parents for percussion and grip myotonia and by electromyographic depiction of myotonic discharges. Duchenne's (pseudohypertrophic) muscular dystrophy clinically appears in children who are about 2 or 3 years of age.

357. The answer is A (1, 2, 3). *(Fishman, pp 171–182.)* When bloody cerebrospinal fluid (CSF) results from a subarachnoid hemorrhage, there will be the same number of red blood cells per mm^3 in the first tube as in the third tube of CSF. With a traumatic lumbar puncture there will be more red blood cells in either the first or the third tube. A lumbar puncture in a higher interspace repeated immediately will be free of blood if the first puncture was traumatic. The supernatant of traumatically bloody CSF will be clear, while that from a CSF with subarachnoid hemorrhage will demonstrate xanthochromia, usually within 2 to 4 hours after the bleeding episode. Because bloody CSF, regardless of cause, rarely clots, observation for clotting will be of no assistance in differentiating the cause.

358. The answer is A (1, 2, 3). *(Menkes, ed 2. pp 55–71.)* The cherry red spot represents the center of a normal retinal macula that is surrounded by ganglion cells in which there is an abnormal accumulation of lipid. This alters the surrounding retinal color so that it is yellowish or grayish white. In the first three disorders noted, there is lipid material in the ganglion cells. Metachromatic leukodystrophy does not affect the retina as it is a demyelinating disorder rather than a "storage" disease.

359. The answer is E (all). *(Volpe, pp 119–124.)* The most frequent causes of neonatal seizures are tetany and birth trauma associated with anoxia. It is not clear in the case of hypocalcemia-related seizures whether the metabolic abnormality acts alone or in addition to brain injury caused by hypoxia to lower the threshold for seizure activity. Anomalies such as porencephaly and agenesis of the corpus callosum may be found in neonates who are having seizures.

360. The answer is E (all). *(Behrman, ed 12. p 1533. Faerø, Epilepsia 13:279–285, 1972. Nelson, N Engl J Med 295:1029–1033, 1976.)* Febrile seizures generally occur in children between the ages of 6 months and 3 years and usually in association with upper respiratory illness, roseola, shigellosis, or gastroenteritis. The generalized seizures are mostly brief (2 to 5 minutes) and the cerebrospinal fluid is normal. Infants who have seizures that are prolonged (longer than 15 minutes), focal, or lateralized or who had neurologic problems before the febrile seizure are at a higher risk than other affected infants for developing an afebrile seizure disorder during the next 5 to 7 years.

361. The answer is E (all). *(Volpe, p 119.)* Jitteriness or rhythmic tremor induced by the stimulation of handling an infant is found in all the listed circumstances. This motor activity can be distinguished from seizures because it is suppressible by flexing the extremity or merely firmly holding it. In addition, in contrast to seizures, this tremulousness is unaccompanied by apnea, eye deviation, or staring. All the circumstances listed may also result in neonatal seizures.

362. The answer is A (1, 2, 3). *(Behrman, ed 12. pp 1575–1576. Swaiman, ed 2. p 790.)* Children who have Sturge-Weber syndrome characteristically can be recognized by the port wine vascular nevus occurring in the distribution of the ophthalmic and maxillary branches of the trigeminal nerve. Angiomas involving the nose, mouth, and lips are not uncommon in these children. Hemiplegia, if present, occurs contralaterally to the port wine stain and leptomeningeal angiomas. Angiomas of the retina, along with cerebellar and spinal cord hemangioblastomas and renal cysts, are characteristic of von Hippel–Lindau disease.

363. The answer is A (1, 2, 3). *(DeVivo, Pediatr Clin North Am 23:527–540, 1976. Pollack, pp 3–14.)* Reye's syndrome should be suspected when a child begins to vomit unremittingly and appears confused, disoriented, or lethargic. This syndrome generally occurs as a child is recovering from a mild viral illness or on the third to fifth day of a chickenpox infection and may be related to concurrent aspirin use. Tachypnea and seizures may develop even in the early stages of the disorder.

The most characteristic laboratory findings are serum transaminase levels at least two times normal, elevated levels of blood ammonia, and prothrombin times that are 2 or more seconds longer than in controls. Hypoglycemia also is common, particularly in younger children. Specific treatment remains controversial, but good supportive care and management of increased intracranial pressure are essential.

364. The answer is A (1, 2, 3). *(Gordon, p 6.)* The most common causes of an asymmetric Moro reflex in infants are injuries to the brachial plexus and clavicular fractures. Humeral, radial, and ulnar fractures also may produce an asymmetric response. Infantile hemiplegia, too, is associated, though less commonly than the factors listed above, with an asymmetric Moro reflex.

365. The answer is A (1,2,3). *(Finberg, p 198.)* Diabetes insipidus is a common complication of severe head trauma and is due to a deficiency in secretion of antidiuretic hormone. It must be distinguished from the polyuria that may occur several days after head injury as the high antidiuretic hormone levels, associated with the head injury, resolve. This form of diabetes insipidus may be treated by replacement of urine losses intravenously or enterally with solutions low in sodium as long as it is possible to keep up with the losses. Vasopressin given intramuscularly or as an intranasal preparation makes care easier and safer as long as water balance is carefully monitored.

Infectious Diseases and Immunology

DIRECTIONS: Each question below contains five suggested responses. Select the **one best** response to each question.

366. All the following viruses have been associated with congenital infections EXCEPT

(A) cytomegalovirus
(B) rubella virus
(C) hepatitis B virus
(D) herpes simplex virus
—(E) rotavirus

367. All the following are recognized complications of chickenpox EXCEPT

(A) Reye's syndrome
(B) encephalitis
(C) pneumonia
(D) hemorrhagic varicella
—(E) orchitis

368. An 8-year-old boy who has no history of sexual contact develops dysuria and a purulent urethral discharge. Culture on chocolate agar shows a few colonies of *Escherichia coli*. Forty-eight hours later, his left ankle becomes swollen, hot, and tender, coincident with the onset of chills, fever, and a stiff neck. A lumbar puncture shows cloudy cerebrospinal fluid. The cause of this disease is most likely to be

— (A) *Neisseria gonorrhoeae*
(B) *Mycoplasma hominis*
(C) T-strain *Mycoplasma*
(D) *Chlamydia*
(E) herpesvirus hominis, type 2

369. A 14-year-old boy is seen in the emergency room because of a 3-week history of fever between 101° and 102°F, lethargy, and a 6-lb weight loss. Physical examination reveals marked cervical and inguinal adenopathy, enlarged tonsils with exudate, and a palpable spleen 2 cm below the left costal margin. The pediatrician suspects infectious mononucleosis. All the following conditions would be consistent with that diagnosis EXCEPT

(A) small hemorrhages on the soft palate
(B) a WBC differential revealing 50 percent lymphocytes and 10 percent atypical lymphocytes
(C) a positive heterophil titer
(D) antibodies to Epstein-Barr virus (EBV) viral capsid antigen at a titer of 1:512
(E) a vesicular exanthem

370. All the following statements about acute osteomyelitis are true EXCEPT that

(A) it most commonly is caused by *Staphylococcus aureus*
(B) it often arises following development of deep cellulitis
(C) tenderness in the region of infection is diffuse, not localized
(D) bony changes are not visible radiographically for 5 to 10 days after onset of infection
(E) antibiotic therapy usually is required for at least 4 weeks

371. A 3-year-old boy has had a temperature of 39°C (102.2°F) and a stiff back for the last 3 days. Examination shows a red throat, large nontender anterior and posterior cervical nodes, and slight resistance of the neck to flexion. Immediate management should include a

(A) lumbar puncture
(B) heterophil test
(C) throat culture and oral penicillin for 7 days
(D) throat culture and oral penicillin for 10 days
(E) throat culture, white blood cell count, and reexamination in 24 hours

372. An 8-day-old infant male with staphylococcal pneumonia is at risk for all the following complications EXCEPT

(A) pneumatocele formation
(B) pneumothorax
(C) empyema
(D) pleural effusion
(E) epiglottitis

373. A 14-month-old infant suddenly develops a fever of 40.2°C (104.4°F). Physical examination shows an alert, active infant who drinks milk eagerly. No physical abnormalities are noted. The white blood cell count is 22,000/mm^3 with 78 percent polymorphonuclear leukocytes, 18 percent of which are band forms. The most likely diagnosis is

(A) pneumococcal bacteremia
(B) roseola
(C) streptococcicosis
(D) typhoid fever
(E) diphtheria

374. The leading cause of bacterial meningitis in children between the ages of 6 months and 3 years is

(A) group A beta-hemolytic strepto-cocci
(B) group C *Neisseria meningitidis*
(C) type 5 *Streptococcus (Diplococcus)* *pneumoniae*
—(D) type B *Haemophilus influenzae*
(E) untypable *Haemophilus influenzae*

375. A 3-year-old child awakens at night with a fever of 39.6°C (103.3°F), a severe sore throat, and a barking cough. Physical examination of the child, who is drooling, shows a very red throat and inspiratory stridor. The hypopharynx is obscured by yellow mucus. There is no respiratory distress. Optimal management would include

— (A) immediate hospitalization for pos-sible intubation
(B) immediate inhalation therapy with racemic epinephrine
(C) treatment with oral ampicillin, 50 mg/kg per day
(D) suctioning of the pharynx and hourly examinations of the hypo-pharynx
(E) a throat culture and initiation of expectorant and mist therapy

376. Which of the following infections typically has an incubation period of less than 2 weeks?

(A) Mumps
(B) Varicella
(C) Rubella
— (D) Measles
(E) Rabies

377. A 14-year-old girl awakens with a mild sore throat, low-grade fever, and a diffuse maculopapular rash. Dur-ing the next 24 hours she develops tender swelling of her wrists and red-ness of her eyes. In addition, her phy-sician notes mild tenderness and marked swelling of her posterior cervi-cal and occipital lymph nodes. Four days after the onset of her illness the rash has vanished.
    The most likely diagnosis of this girl's condition is

— (A) rubella
(B) rubeola
(C) roseola
(D) erythema infectiosum
(E) erythema multiforme

378. A 5-year-old boy develops a mild sore throat, malaise, a low-grade fever, and a faint, generalized, rough, fine red papular rash most obvious on the trunk. His tongue is coated as shown in figure A below. After 3 days the rash has faded, and his tongue appears as in figure B. One week later there is a sudden, alarming loss of the superficial layers of skin from his fingers.

The most likely diagnosis of this child's condition is

(A) rubella
(B) erythema infectiosum (fifth disease)
(C) roseola
(D) scarlet fever
(E) thrush

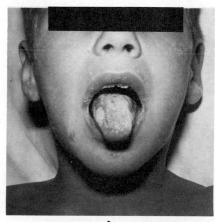

A

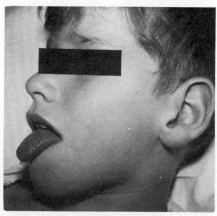

B

379. Rocky Mountain spotted fever is an acute illness characterized by fever, muscle pain, and a rash that is most prominent on the extremities. The disease is caused by *Rickettsia rickettsii,* which is transmitted by the bite of a tick. All the following would be characteristic in a patient with this diagnosis EXCEPT

(A) a history of a tick bite 9 days prior to presentation
(B) a maculopapular rash that began on the flexor surfaces of the wrist
(C) evolution of the rash to a hemorrhagic appearance
(D) a low serum sodium associated with thrombocytopenia
(E) a purulent tonsillitis

380. Rocky Mountain spotted fever must always be considered when a child from an endemic area presents with fever and a rash on the extremities. Other possibilities that should be considered in the differential diagnosis of Rocky Mountain spotted fever include all the following EXCEPT

(A) a petechial rash caused by *Neisseria meningitidis*
(B) viral infections
(C) atypical measles
(D) toxic shock syndrome
(E) varicella

381. The rash and mucous membrane lesions shown below develop in an infant 5 days after a nonspecific upper respiratory tract infection. Which of the following is LEAST likely to be responsible?

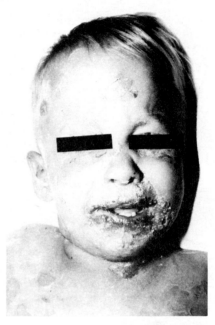

(A) *Mycoplasma pneumoniae*
(B) Herpesvirus hominis, type 1
(C) Rubella virus
(D) Phenobarbital ingestion
(E) Penicillin therapy

382. Which of the following statements about aplastic anemia caused by chloramphenicol therapy is correct?

(A) It occurs in about 0.01 percent of those receiving the therapy
(B) It is usually dose-related
(C) It disappears when treatment is discontinued
(D) It appears during therapy rather than after therapy
(E) None of the above

383. Streptococcal pyoderma (impetigo) is best described as

(A) a vesicular or bullous infection in which the blisters rupture over a period of many hours

(B) a vesicular infection in which blisters rupture early and crusts develop

(C) a vesicular infection characterized by painful, brown, crusted lesions that spread out on the face

(D) a vesicular infection producing painful, indurated, thick-walled vesicles on a red fingertip

(E) a vesicular infection in which painful vesicles are arranged in a linear pattern

384. The organisms most frequently found in middle ear fluid in patients with otitis media are

(A) viruses

(B) fungi

(C) bacteria resistant to ampicillin

(D) bacteria sensitive to ampicillin

(E) algae

DIRECTIONS: Each question below contains four suggested responses of which **one or more** is correct. Select

A	if	**1, 2, and 3**	are correct
B	if	**1 and 3**	are correct
C	if	**2 and 4**	are correct
D	if	**4**	is correct
E	if	**1, 2, 3, and 4**	are correct

385. True statements regarding infant botulism include which of the following?

(1) A distinct prodrome consisting of constipation, poor feeding, weak cry, and loss of head control is often seen

(2) In infant botulism, the preformed toxin is contained in food ingested by the infant

(3) Findings on physical examination include diffuse hypotonia, weak suck, and absent deep tendon reflexes

(4) Most infants never show a complete resolution of symptoms

386. Twelve hours after eating her Christmas dinner, a 3-year-old girl develops vomiting, abdominal cramps, low-grade fever, and profuse watery diarrhea that fails to improve with a clear liquid diet. Stool cultures obtained on the fourth day because of persistent diarrhea show neither *Salmonella* nor *Shigella* species. However, additional studies might be expected to show

(1) *Yersinia enterocolitica*
(2) a rotavirus infection
(3) *Campylobacter fetus*
(4) *Clostridium difficile*

387. A newborn infant has an abnormally small head; a skull x-ray is shown below. The radiographic findings are characteristic of infection with which of the following organisms?

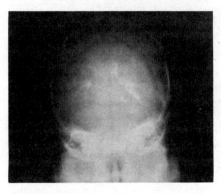

(1) *Toxoplasma gondii*
(2) *Treponema pallidum*
(3) Cytomegalovirus
(4) Rubella virus

388. Infectious mononucleosis is a disease caused by the Epstein-Barr virus (EBV). A patient with this disease usually has a triad of findings consisting of the appropriate changes in physical examination, the associated serologic changes, and the corresponding hematologic abnormalities. True statements about infectious mononucleosis include which of the following?

—(1) The incubation period is 4 to 6 weeks
— (2) Fifteen percent of seropositive individuals excrete virus at any one point
— (3) Transmission of the disease is mainly via saliva containing EBV; thus, epidemics do not occur
(4) A person may be infected by an exogenous strain of EBV on more than one occasion

389. A 15-year-old boy returned to his pediatrician because of a persistent, but moderately improved, urethral discharge 2 weeks following treatment with intramuscular procaine penicillin G, 4.8 million units, and oral probenecid, 1 g. A Gram stain of the original discharge had shown many gram-negative diplococci within abundant leukocytes. When reexamined, no organisms could be identified either by stain or bacteriologic culture. Manifestations of disease in other individuals infected with the boy's persistent pathogen or with related serotypes would be likely to include

(1) persistent tachypnea, cough, and inspiratory rales in a 2-month-old infant
(2) purulent conjunctival discharge in a 3-day-old infant
— (3) fever and tender swollen inguinal lymph nodes
(4) lobar pneumonia in a 16-year-old girl

390. A newborn infant becomes markedly jaundiced on the second day of life, and a faint petechial eruption first noted at birth is now a generalized purpuric rash. Hematologic studies for hemolytic diseases are negative. Appropriate measures at this time would include

—(1) radiographic examination of the long bones
— (2) isolation of the infant from pregnant hospital personnel
— (3) a blood culture
— (4) measurement of the level of serum immunoglobulin M

391. Common features of infections with hepatitis A virus include which of the following?

(1) Prolonged presence of virus in stools

(2) Short incubation period (15 to 50 days)

(3) Frequent occurrence of extrahepatic manifestations

(4) Sudden onset of fever, nausea, and vomiting

392. It has been estimated that during the period 1977–1978 there were between 5 and 10 million deaths worldwide caused by acute infectious diarrhea. The precise role played by viral gastroenteritis is not clear, although it is safe to state that rotaviruses and the Norwalk-like viruses play an important role. True statements about rotaviruses include which of the following?

(1) The name of the virus is derived from the Latin word rota, which means "wheel," because in the electron microscope the virus particle resembles the rim of a wheel connected by short spokes

(2) Rotavirus is the major pathogen in infantile gastroenteritis

(3) Rotaviral diarrhea is characterized by watery stools with fever and vomiting and isotonic dehydration

(4) Adults are rarely infected by rotavirus

393. A 2-month-old infant has a temperature of 39.6°C (103.3°F); physical examination is completely normal. Which of the following types of infection should be considered in the diagnostic evaluation?

(1) Roseola infantum

(2) Bacterial meningitis

(3) Streptococcal pharyngitis

(4) Urinary tract infection

394. In addition to the familiar maculopapular rash, measles typically is characterized by which of the following symptoms?

(1) Cough

(2) Moderate or high fever

(3) Coryza

(4) Conjunctivitis

395. Correct statements about disease caused by *Candida albicans* include which of the following?

(1) *Candida albicans* may be found in the intestinal tract and on the mucous membranes of normal individuals as a yeast form

(2) Systemic disease caused by *Candida* occurs primarily in individuals who are immunocompromised, have diabetes mellitus, or have received antibiotics and corticosteroids

(3) Chronic mucocutaneous candidiasis is a syndrome associated with defects in T-cell immunity

(4) There is no effective therapy for disseminated disease caused by *Candida*

396. A positive Mantoux test in a child may

- (1) develop within 2 to 10 weeks after infection
- (2) indicate infection with atypical mycobacteria
- (3) indicate a need for antimicrobial therapy
- (4) become negative for a brief period after immunization with live viruses

397. A 3-year-old black male with known sickle cell anemia developed a painful, tender swelling of his foot, accompanied by a temperature of 39°C (102.2°F). His white blood cell count was 10,600/mm^3 (72 percent polymorphonuclear leukocytes and 18 percent lymphocytes), and his erythrocyte sedimentation rate was 56 mm per hour. An x-ray of his foot is shown below. True statements about this child's illness include which of the following?

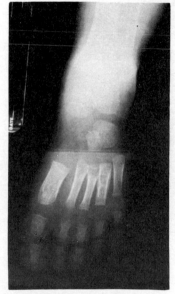

Courtesy of Donald Darling, M.D.

- (1) *Salmonella* organisms may be found in his blood
- (2) His sodium metabisulfite blood test is likely to be abnormal
- (3) Polyvalent pneumococcal vaccine may significantly reduce his future morbidity
- (4) Intravenous penicillin is the treatment of choice

400. Meningococcemia can lead to which of the following complications?

—(1) Acute adrenal failure
—(2) Arthritis
— (3) Gastrointestinal hemorrhage
— (4) Pericarditis

398. A 10-year-old boy from the Connecticut coast is seen because of discomfort in his right knee. He had a large annular erythematous lesion on his back that disappeared 4 weeks prior to the present visit. His mother recalls pulling a tick off his back. Correct statements about this child's likely illness include which of the following?

—(1) The skin lesion is called erythema chronicum migrans
— (2) The disease is caused by a spirochete that is transmitted by the bite of a tick
—(3) In addition to skin and joint involvement, CNS and cardiac abnormalities may be present
— (4) Penicillin therapy results in a more rapid resolution of symptoms than occurs in untreated patients

401. Disease is produced by which of the following parasites in the course of their migration through the parenchyma of body tissues?

— (1) *Necator americanus*
—(2) *Ascaris lumbricoides*
—(3) *Toxocara canis*
(4) *Enterobius vermicularis*

399. True statements about poliomyelitis include which of the following?

—(1) It can be asymptomatic or nonparalytic
—(2) It is accompanied by fever, sore throat, and myalgia
—(3) Aseptic meningitis can be a prominent feature
— (4) Hypertension and urinary retention sometimes arise as complications

402. A newborn infant has the desqua-
mating rash depicted in the figure below. The child might also be expected
to develop which of the following conditions?

(1) Purulent umbilical drainage
(2) Pneumonia
(3) Progressive enlargement of one
breast
(4) An asymmetric Moro reflex

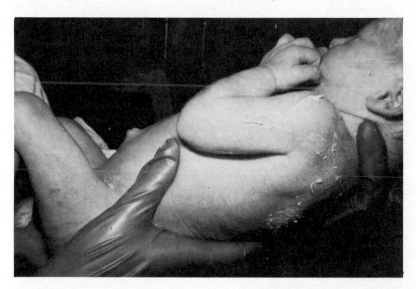

403. A child who has croup can be expected to

(1) have a low-grade fever
(2) wheeze during expiration
(3) be infected with parainfluenza virus
(4) show hyperinflation on chest x-ray

404. Complications of otitis media include

(1) cholesteatoma
(2) mastoiditis
(3) Gradenigo's syndrome
(4) brain abscess

405. Two weeks ago, a 5-year-old boy developed diarrhea, which has persisted to the present time in spite of dietary management. His stools have been watery, pale, and frothy. He has been afebrile. Microscopic examination of his stools might show

(1) *Trichuris trichiura*
(2) *Entamoeba histolytica*
(3) *Giardia lamblia*
(4) *Toxoplasma gondii*

DIRECTIONS: Each group of questions below consists of lettered headings followed by a set of numbered items. For each numbered item select the **one** lettered heading with which it is **most** closely associated. Each lettered heading may be used **once, more than once, or not at all.**

Questions 406–407

For each of the phagocytic disorders described below, select the syndrome or disease with which it is most closely associated.

(A) Lazy leukocyte syndrome
(B) Chediak-Higashi syndrome
(C) Chronic granulomatous disease
(D) Ataxia-telangiectasia
(E) None of the above

406. Abscesses, pneumonia, and osteomyelitis accompany this sex-linked or autosomal recessive condition in which leukocytes manifest normal attachment and phagocytosis but are not microbicidal for catalase-positive organisms because of defective oxidative metabolism

407. Recurrent, severe bacterial and viral infections occur in this neutropenic disorder in which leukocytes demonstrate defective chemotaxis, delayed degranulation of giant lysosomes, and normal, but delayed, intracellular killing

Questions 408–411

For each of the immunologic abnormalities listed in the table below, select the syndrome or disease with which it is most closely associated.

(A) Bruton's disease
(B) Di George's syndrome
(C) Wiskott-Aldrich syndrome
(D) Job-Buckley syndrome
(E) Swiss-type immunodeficiency disease (severe combined immunodeficiency disease [SCID])

	Serum IgG	Serum IgA	Serum IgM	T-Cell Function	Parathyroid Function
408.	Normal	Normal	Normal	Decreased	Decreased
409.	Low	Low	Low	Normal	Normal
410.	Low	Low	Low	Decreased	Normal
411.	Normal	High	Low	Decreased	Normal

Infectious Diseases and Immunology

Answers

366. The answer is E. *(Behrman, ed 12. pp 399–403, 412–415.)* Rubella virus still causes congenital infections in the United States. Outbreaks occur among young adults, and there is some evidence that the number of susceptible women of child-bearing age is increasing. Cytomegalovirus (CMV) is a major cause of congenital disease in this country. With 50 percent of those pregnant women who experience a primary infection, fetal infection will occur. Approximately 10 percent of these infants will develop some form of damage, such as intrauterine growth retardation, microcephaly, or deafness. The incidence of herpes neonatorum seems to be increasing in parallel with the increase in genital herpes in the United States today. The virus becomes disseminated in two thirds of infected infants, involving the liver, adrenals, and central nervous system. The fatality rate from herpes simplex virus infection of the newborn approaches 80 percent in untreated infants. Hepatitis B virus may be transmitted to the fetus via the transplacental route or to the newborn by close contact with an infectious adult. Of those viruses mentioned, only rotavirus has not been shown to cause congenital disease.

367. The answer is E. *(Rudolph, ed 17. p 612.)* All the complications listed in the question may be associated with chickenpox except for orchitis. Inflammation of the gonads is primarily associated with infection by rubella and mumps virus. Reye's syndrome is also a recognized complication of influenza and has been associated with the use of aspirin for these infections. Varicella encephalitis occurs in less than 1 per 1000 cases of varicella. Typically, the encephalitis involves inflammation of the cerebellum. Symptoms usually begin within 1 week following the onset of the exanthem. Varicella pneumonia may be due to direct involvement of the lung parenchyma by the varicella virus, particularly in adults, or secondary to bacterial infection. Pneumonia as a complication of varicella has a variable course. Symptoms may be minimal or the pneumonia may be an early sign of disseminated infection. Hemorrhagic varicella is a rare complication of chickenpox and is characterized by high-grade fever and hemorrhage into the vesicles.

368. The answer is A. *(Behrman, ed 12. pp 653–655. Handsfield, N Engl J Med 306:950–954, 1982. Krugman, ed 7. pp 77–89. Taylor-Robinson, N Engl J Med 302:1003–1010, 1063–1067, 1980.)* If vaginal or urethral discharge is present, gonococcal infection must be suspected, regardless of the affected individual's age or sexual history. The Laboratory demonstration of *Neisseria gonorrhoeae* is usually but not always possible using both a Gram stain of the exudate and a culture on Thayer-Martin medium, which is more selective than chocolate agar. Gonococci can spread either hematogenously or by direct extension; infection can cause inflammation or abscess formation in the epididymis, prostate gland, fallopian tubes, peritoneal cavity, liver, and joints. Gonococcal endocarditis or meningitis, though rare, occasionally can develop. Nongonococcal urethritis accompanied by dysuria and purulent discharge, once attributed to T-stain mycoplasmas, is now thought to be caused mainly by species of *Chlamydia*. However, although this infection may be complicated by arthritis and conjunctivitis (Reiter's syndrome), meningitis does not occur. Most authorities no longer acknowledge *Mycoplasma hominis* to be a cause of symptomatic urethritis. The genital strain (type 2) of herpesvirus hominis produces a painful vesiculating balanitis or vulvitis.

Treatment of gonococcal infections has traditionally included penicillin therapy. However, since the first description in 1976 of penicillinase-producing strains of *N. gonorrhoeae*, careful patient follow-up has been necessary to ensure adequate therapy. Although the incidence of penicillin-resistant gonococci is low, localized outbreaks caused by resistant strains have been described in several urban areas. Resistant strains of *N. gonorrhoeae* are generally treated with either spectinomycin or newer generation cephalosporins.

369. The answer is E. *(Rudolph, ed 17. pp 592–594.)* A vesicular exanthem is not characteristic of infectious mononucleosis. To prove a diagnosis of infectious mononucleosis, a triad of findings should be present. First, physical findings may include diffuse adenopathy, tonsilar enlargement, an enlarged spleen, small hemorrhages on the soft palate, and periorbital swelling. Second, the hematologic changes should reveal a predominance of lymphocytes with at least 10 percent of these cells being atypical. Third, the characteristic antibody response should be present. Traditionally, heterophil antibodies can be detected when confirming a diagnosis of infectious mononucleosis. However, these antibodies may not be present, particularly in young children. Alternatively, specific antibodies against viral capsid antigen (VCA) on the Epstein-Barr virus may be measured. A titer of 1:152 suggests either a past infection or a recent exposure with a rising titer. Although a rash may be seen in patients with infectious mononucleosis, a vesicular exanthem is unlikely.

370. The answer is C. *(Behrman, ed 12. pp 613–615. Fleischer, Am J Dis Child 134:499–502, 1980.)* Acute osteomyelitis tends to begin abruptly with fever and marked, localized bone tenderness that usually occurs at the metaphysis. Redness and swelling frequently follow. Although usually the result of hematogenous bacterial spread, particularly of *Staphylococcus aureus*, acute osteomyelitis may follow an episode of deep cellulitis and should be suspected whenever deep cellulitis occurs. Diagnosis must often be based on clinical grounds, because bone changes may not be visible on x-ray for up to 12 days after onset of the disease. However, bone scans with technetium radioisotopes may be useful in the early diagnosis of osteomyelitis and in its differentiation from cellulitis and septic arthritis. Caution must be exercised, however, when interpreting a normal bone scan in a patient suspected of having osteomyelitis. It is clear that falsely normal bone scans do occur in patients with active bone infection. Antibiotic treatment must be initiated immediately to avoid further extension of infection into bone, where adequate drug levels are difficult to achieve. Treatment is usually continued for at least 4 weeks. In addition to x-rays and white blood cell count, erythrocyte sedimentation rate is useful in monitoring a patient's recovery.

371. The answer is A. *(Behrman, ed 12. p 621. Dodge, N Engl J Med 272:954–960, 1003–1010, 1965.)* A fever accompanied by inability to flex rather than rotate the neck immediately suggests meningitis. An indolent clinical course does not rule out bacterial meningitis: *Haemophilus influenzae* may produce meningeal symptoms (fever, headache, and stiff neck or back) that are so mild that several days can elapse before medical advice is sought. The large cervical nodes characteristic of streptococcal pharyngitis may limit rotational or lateral neck movement if their tenderness is exacerbated by contraction of the sternocleidomastoid muscles. Initial symptoms of infectious mononucleosis with associated aseptic meningitis usually are pharyngitis, adenopathy (often nontender), and meningeal signs. A lumbar puncture is of prime diagnostic importance in determining the presence of bacterial meningitis, which requires immediate antibiotic therapy. A delay in treatment of even 1 hour may lead to such complications as cerebrovascular thrombosis, obstructive hydrocephalus, cerebritis with seizures or acute increased intracranial pressure, coma, or death.

372. The answer is E. *(Behrman, ed 12. pp 1050–1052.)* Staphylococcal pneumonia is a disease seen in patients at both ends of the age spectrum. Staphylococcal pneumonia may occur as a primary infection of the lung or as a complication of a number of viral infections such as measles, chickenpox, or influenza. Illness generally begins as an upper respiratory tract infection without specific features. The illness often progresses rapidly with the sudden onset of high fever, tachypnea, and dyspnea. Pneumatocele formation is characteristic of staphylococcal pneumonia, although it may be seen in pneumonia caused by the pneumococcus or by *Haemophilus influenzae*. Pneumothorax results when there is a rupture of a pneumatocele. Empyema results when the infection escapes the parenchyma of the lung and extends into the pleural cavity. Epiglottitis is not caused by the staphylococcus.

373. The answer is A. *(Behrman, ed 12. pp 612–613, 634. Feder, Clin Pediatr 19:457–462, 1980.)* In an infant who appears otherwise normal, the sudden onset of high fever together with a marked elevation and shift to the left of the white blood cell count suggests pneumococcal bacteremia. Viral infections such as roseola seldom cause such profound shifts in the blood leukocyte count. Streptococcicosis refers to prolonged, low-grade, insidious nasopharyngitis that sometimes occurs in infants infected with group A beta-hemolytic streptococci. Neither typhoid fever nor diphtheria produces markedly high white blood cell counts; both are characterized by headache, malaise, and other systemic signs. Other bacteria that should be considered in a child with this presentation include *H. influenzae* type B and the meningococcus.

374. The answer is D. *(Behrman, ed 12. p 656.)* Haemophilus influenzae, in a nonencapsulated, untypable form, can cause chronic lung disease and acute otitis media. Encapsulated strains are typed A through F, with type B being responsible for almost all the serious infections—including meningitis, pneumonia, bacteremia, and epiglottitis—caused by this organism. The incidence of these infections increases at about the age of 6 months, when levels of passively transferred maternal antibody and opsonins decline, and decreases at about 5 years of age, presumably following repeated infections with this organism. Epidemiologic data from the Center for Disease Control for the years 1977 through 1981 indicate the main percentages of causes of bacterial meningitis in the United States to be as follows: *H. influenzae,* 43 percent; *N. meningitidis,* 27 percent; and *S. pneumoniae,* 11 percent.

375. The answer is A. *(Behrman, ed 12. pp 656–657, 1034–1035.)* Children who have acute epiglottitis, a life-threatening infection of the hypopharynx and epiglottis caused by *Haemophilus influenzae,* typically present with high fever, extremely sore throat, and a croupy cough. Physical examination characteristically shows a red throat and a red, swollen epiglottis that may be obscured by exudate or so distorted that its identity is misinterpreted. It is important that caution be exercised while attempting to visualize the epiglottis. Abrupt glottic spasm is a well-recognized, potentially fatal complication in these patients. Affected children often are unable to swallow saliva, and because the swollen epiglottis can unpredictably and suddenly cause total and fatal airway obstruction, immediate hospitalization is mandatory, even in the absence of severe respiratory distress. If a diagnosis of acute epiglottitis is uncertain, a lateral x-ray of the neck will differentiate epiglottic from subglottic swelling, the latter being associated with a less serious disease, viral croup.

376. The answer is D. *(AAP-CID, ed 20. pp 235, 248, 294, 311, 400.)* The usual incubation periods of several important diseases are as follows: measles, 8 to 12 days; varicella, 14 to 16 days; rubella, 16 to 18 days; mumps, 16 to 18 days; and rabies, 9 days to several months. The durations of infectivity are as follows: measles, from 2 days before the onset of the catarrhal stage through the fifth day of the rash; varicella, from 2 days before the eruption until the last vesicle has dried (approximately 7 days); rubella, from 7 days before the onset of the rash to up to 14 days after its onset (infants with congenital rubella may excrete the virus for more than 1 year); mumps, from 7 days before until 9 days after the onset of parotid swelling.

377. The answer is A. *(Behrman, ed 12. pp 747–751, 1680–1681.)* Symptoms of rubella, usually a mild disease, include a diffuse maculopapular rash that lasts for 3 days, marked enlargement of the posterior cervical and occipital lymph nodes, low-grade fever, mild sore throat, and, occasionally, conjunctivitis, arthralgia, or arthritis. Individuals who have rubeola develop a severe cough, coryza, photophobia, conjunctivitis, and a high fever that reaches its peak at the height of the generalized macular rash, which typically lasts for 5 days; Koplik's spots on the buccal mucosa are diagnostic. Roseola is a viral exanthem of infants in which the high fever abruptly abates as a rash appears. Erythema infectiosum (fifth disease) begins with bright erythema on the cheeks ("slapped cheek" sign), followed by a red maculopapular rash on the trunk and extremities, which fades centrally at first. Erythema multiforme is a poorly understood syndrome consisting of skin lesions and mucous membrane involvement. A number of infectious agents and drugs have been associated with this syndrome.

378. The answer is D. *(Behrman, ed 12. pp 634–635.)* Scarlet fever results when group A beta-hemolytic streptococci infecting the throat or other sites produce an erythrogenic toxin that acutely inflames the skin, kidneys, joints, or heart. The disease is easily identified by the following features: a primary site of bacterial infection, usually in the throat; a generalized, fine papular rash that has a "sandpaper" texture, is worse in the skin creases, and often involves the tongue, on which red papillae project above a thick white coat (strawberry tongue); and, following the rash, desquamation of branlike scales especially from the fingers and the tongue, causing the latter to appear red and denuded (raspberry tongue). Scarlet fever is one of the fascinating diseases that have clearly undergone a change in epidemiology and in severity in recent years. Whereas scarlet fever was formerly associated with severe sequelae, the majority of cases today are mild.

379. The answer is E. *(Rudolph, ed 17. pp 643–644.)* The incubation period for Rocky Mountain spotted fever has a range of 3 to 12 days. A brief prodromal period consisting of headache and malaise is typically followed by the abrupt onset of fever and chills. A maculopapular rash starts on the third or fourth day of illness on the flexor surfaces of the wrists and ankles before moving in a central direction. Typically, the palms and soles are involved. The rash may become hemorrhagic within 1 or 2 days. Hyponatremia and thrombocytopenia may be seen. A purulent pharyngitis is not characteristic.

380. The answer is E. *(Rudolph, ed 17. pp 625, 643, 644.)* Varicella is not generally confused with Rocky Mountain spotted fever. A morbilliform eruption may precede a petechial rash caused by *Neisseria meningitidis*. In addition, septic shock is a common complication of meningococcemia. Viral infections, particularly the enteroviruses, may cause a severe illness that resembles Rocky Mountain spotted fever. In addition, several viruses have been associated with disseminated intravascular coagulation. Atypical measles is seen primarily in children who received the killed measles vaccine before 1968. After exposure to wild type measles, such a person may develop a prodrome consisting of fever, cough, headache, and myalgia. This is usually followed by the development of pneumonia and an urticarial rash beginning on the extremities. Toxic shock syndrome (TSS) is a disease characterized by sudden onset of fever, diarrhea, shock, mucous membrane inflammation, and a diffuse macular rash resulting in desquamation of the hands and feet. Fluid loss with shock is a common complication. TSS occurs most commonly in menstruating women and appears to be associated with the presence of a toxin-producing strain of *S. aureus* in the vagina.

381. The answer is C. *(Behrman, ed 12. p 584.)* The combination of erythema multiforme and vesicular, ulcerated lesions of the mucous membranes of the eyes, mouth, anus, and urethra defines the Stevens-Johnson syndrome (erythema multiforme exudativum). Fever is common and pulmonary involvement occasionally is noted; the mortality can approach 10 percent. Common complications include corneal ulceration, dehydration owing to severe stomatitis and subsequently poor fluid intake, and urinary retention caused by dysuria. Among the known causes of the Stevens-Johnson syndrome are allergy to various drugs (including barbiturates, sulfonamides, and penicillin) and infection with *Mycoplasma pneumoniae*.

382. The answer is E. *(Meissner, Pediatrics 64:348–356, 1976.)* Aplastic anemia induced by chloramphenicol is relatively uncommon (1 case in every 60,000 to 100,000 individuals receiving the drug). It has been estimated that the incidence of chloramphenicol-induced aplastic anemia is about the same as that of death caused by penicillin anaphylaxis. Not usually related to dose, it is an idiosyncratic reaction that can occur either during therapy or up to many months after; it usually has a fatal outcome. In contrast, chloramphenicol-induced bone marrow suppression is extremely common, is related to dose, occurs during therapy, and responds satisfactorily to a reduction in dose or cessation of treatment.

383. The answer is B. *(Behrman, ed 12. pp 752, 758–759, 1711–1712. Dillon, Am J Dis Child 115:530–541, 1968. Peter, N Engl J Med 297:311–317, 1977.)* Streptococcal impetigo is a superficial pyoderma in which thin-walled vesicles rupture very rapidly, creating oozing or crusted honey-colored sores; these sores may be the first lesions noted by an affected individual. The vesicles of staphylococcal impetigo are more durable and may not rupture as the lesions spread. Impetigo is usually painless; painful, crusted, spreading lesions on the face are ordinarily caused by herpesvirus hominis, type 1, which also can cause a distinctive, painful, red swelling of a fingertip with clusters of thick wall vesicles. Herpes zoster infection features painful vesicles in a linear arrangement along dermatomes. Staphylococcal impetigo most frequently develops in neonates in the periumbilical area, whereas impetigo contagiosa is primarily an endemic disease of children under school age.

384. The answer is D. *(Behrman, ed 12. pp 1026–1027.)* *Streptococcus pneumoniae* and *Haemophilus influenzae* are the most common organisms found in otitis media. They are generally sensitive to ampicillin and amoxacillin, which are the drugs of first choice in treating a patient not allergic to them. *Haemophilus influenzae* is developing increasing resistance to ampicillin and amoxacillin and when there is poor response to initial treatment, trimethoprim-sulfamethoxazole, erythromycin-sulfonamide combinations, or a cephalosporin may be tried.

385. The answer is B (1, 3). *(Thompson, Pediatrics 66:936–942, 1980.)* Infant botulism is a neuromuscular disease caused by the toxin of *Clostridium botulinum*. The disease is distinct from classic botulism in that spores are ingested and the toxin is synthesized by the organism while it resides in the infant's intestine. The toxin is then absorbed and produces weakness and paralysis because of impaired release of acetylcholine at the neuromuscular synapse. Recent evidence suggests a broad clinical spectrum of infant botulism. Some infants may never require hospitalization and demonstrate only minimal feeding difficulties. More severely affected infants may have a presentation that suggests the sudden infant death syndrome. Infants who survive show a complete resolution of symptoms.

386. The answer is A (1, 2, 3). *(Kohl, Pediatr Clin North Am 26:433–443, 1979. Prince, Pediatr Clin North Am 26:261–268, 1979. Steinhoff, J Pediatr 96:611–622, 1980. Torphy, Pediatrics 64:898–903, 1979.)* *Yersinia enterocolitica* is a gram-negative, invasive member of the Enterobacteriaceae family. As the etiologic agent of one form of prolonged diarrhea, with vomiting, fever, and abdominal pain that may resemble acute appendicitis, it is rarely identified by routine bacteriologic cultures. Because it can be isolated easily with special bacteriologic techniques, some authorities predict that *Y. enterocolitica* will prove to be an important cause of common-source outbreaks of gastroenteritis. Human rotavirus infection is characterized by winter outbreaks of sudden vomiting, fever, and diarrhea, often accompanied by upper respiratory tract symptoms. It may affect both adults and children within families and appears to be the single most important etiologic agent in childhood gastroenteritis. *Campylobacter fetus* (formerly *Vibrio fetus*) is emerging as an important cause of both common-source and sporadic diarrhea. The enteritis commonly is associated with severe abdominal cramps and diarrheal stools, which may contain blood or mucus. In addition to enteritis, at least two other patterns of human disease occur with infection with this pathogen: bacteremia and focal infections in older, debilitated men, and perinatal infections of mothers or infants. Special bacteriologic techniques are required to isolate this organism. During either oral or parenteral therapy with antibiotics, particularly ampicillin, penicillin, and clindamycin, the normal bowel flora are markedly reduced in number, allowing proliferation of *Clostridium difficile*. These bacteria elaborate a toxin, which then produces profuse watery diarrhea, fever, vomiting, and abdominal distension, with typical pseudomembranous plaques visible by proctoscopy. This syndrome, known as antibiotic-associated pseudomembranous colitis, usually remits when the antibiotic is stopped but may in some cases progress to toxic megacolon, peritonitis, and shock. In such cases, intravenous fluid replacement and eradication of the clostridia with vancomycin may be lifesaving.

387. The answer is B (1, 3). *(Krugman, ed 7. pp 4–8, 417–425.)* Microcephaly accompanied by intracranial calcification is highly characteristic of congenital toxoplasmosis or infection with cytomegalovirus. Definitive diagnosis of either disease may be made by demonstration of a rising antibody titer to either pathogen; in addition, cytomegalovirus can be cultured from the urine of affected individuals. It is important to note that maternal immunoglobulin G antibodies may passively cross the placenta and initially produce positive serologic titers in the newborn for *Toxoplasma, Treponema,* cytomegalovirus, or rubella. Therefore, to document that an antibody is of fetal origin, a stable or rising antibody titer must be demonstrated or the nondiffusible immunoglobulin M antibody fraction must be tested.

388. The answer is A (1, 2, 3). *(Sullivan, Adv Pediatr 31:365–399, 1984.)* The Epstein-Barr virus has one of the longest incubation periods of any conventional virus. Once an individual has been infected by the Epstein-Barr virus, the virus is carried in B lymphocytes for the life of the host. Periodically, the virus is excreted from B lymphocytes into the saliva of the infected host. At any one point, 15 percent of seropositive individuals will excrete the virus in their saliva. When a seronegative individual comes in contact with saliva containing EBV; primary infection may occur. Once a person has had a primary EBV infection, a fresh infection by an exogenous virus does not occur. However, there may be reactivation of the endogenous Epstein-Barr virus infection under certain circumstances when the latent virus is permitted to reactivate.

389. The answer is B (1, 3). *(Lumicao, Pediatr Clin North Am 26:269–282, 1979. Tipple, Pediatrics 63:192–197, 1979.)* Chlamydial species include *Chlamydia psittaci* and *Chlamydia trachomatis,* both of which are pathogenic for humans. *C. psittaci* causes ornithosis, an infection ordinarily contracted from birds, principally parrots, parakeets, turkeys, and ducks. Ornithosis is characterized by interstitial pneumonia, fever, headache, and myalgias. Much more prevalent are infections with various serotypes of *C. trachomatis,* which cause trachoma, chlamydial conjunctivitis of the newborn, chlamydial pneumonia of infancy, nongonococcal and postgonococcal urethritis, and lymphogranuloma venereum. Chlamydial conjunctivitis of the newborn (inclusion blenorrhea) can be differentiated from other causes of neonatal conjunctivitis by the time of onset and by culture and stain techniques. In contrast to the chemical conjunctivitis produced by silver nitrate eye drops, which occurs within the first 2 days of life, and to bacterial conjunctivitis, which often develops within the first week of life and can be identified with routine bacteriologic cultures and Gram stain, inclusion blenorrhea typically appears at approximately 10 to 14 days of life. The characteristic inclusion bodies may be seen within the cytoplasm of epithelial cells obtained by conjunctival swabbing and Giemsa staining. Chlamydial pneumonia of infancy usually occurs between 1 and 3 months of age and develops gradually. Characterized clinically by a frequent and persistent cough, tachypnea, inspiratory rales, normal temperature, and a chest x-ray pattern of interstitial infiltrates and hyperinflation, the illness tends to continue for several weeks. Lymphogranuloma venereum (LGV) is a sexually transmitted disease caused by three relatively invasive serotypes of *C. trachomatis*. Following the production of a primary lesion on the genitals or urethra, a second stage occurs, with tender enlargement of the regional lymph nodes, often accompanied by a fever. A third stage, with tissue destruction leading to rectal strictures, may occur.

390. The answer is E (all). *(Behrman, ed 12. pp 399–401, 411–413, 848. Krugman, ed 7. pp 7–8, 322–326, 395–399, 421–423.)* Sepsis of the newborn may first manifest as jaundice and thrombocytopenic purpura. Among the important causes of neonatal sepsis are prenatal infections, including congenital syphilis, toxoplasmosis, cytomegalic inclusion disease, and rubella. Useful diagnostic studies, in addition to cultures for bacteria, include specific serologic tests for pathogens, viral cultures for cytomegalovirus, lumbar puncture, x-rays of the chest and long bones, and measurement of the cord-blood immunoglobulin M level, which often is increased in prenatal infections. Longitudinal striations in the metaphyses are characteristic of congenital rubella, while osteochondritis or periostitis usually indicates congenital syphilis. Congenital syphilis, cytomegalovirus disease, and rubella may be highly contagious. Urine may contain rubella virus for more than 6 months and is therefore a special hazard to nonimmune pregnant women.

391. The answer is C (2, 4). *(AAP-CID, ed 20. pp 178–189. Seto, Pediatr Clin North Am 26:305–314, 1979.)* Hepatitis A (infectious hepatitis) is characterized by a relatively short incubation period (15 to 50 days) following transmission of the virus, primarily by the fecal-oral route. Its onset is abrupt, with sudden fever, nausea, vomiting, anorexia, and liver tenderness, soon followed by jaundice. Elevated serum levels of bilirubin and aspartate aminotransferase (glutamic-oxaloacetic transaminase, SGOT) are transient, usually not persisting more than 3 weeks. Viremia is brief and the period of maximum infectivity of stools usually occurs during the 2-week period prior to the onset of jaundice. Hepatitis B (serum hepatitis), usually transmitted parenterally via blood or blood products, may also be transmitted nonparenterally via body fluids such as saliva or semen. Following a long incubation period (40 to 180 days), there is gradual onset of low fever, anorexia, and jaundice, often preceded or accompanied by extrahepatic manifestations such as macular rashes, arthralgias, or urticaria, which may mimic serum sickness. Serum levels of SGOT and bilirubin may be elevated for months, the latter sometimes rising to levels greater than 20 mg per 100 ml when associated with the fulminant hepatitis more often seen with hepatitis B infection. Viremia usually persists throughout the clinical course of hepatitis B infections and may progress to a chronic carrier state in 10 percent of individuals, most of whom are asymptomatic. These may be identified by the persistence of the viral surface antigen HB_s Ag in their blood. A third type of hepatitis is referred to as non-A, non-B hepatitis, which is important because it accounts for 80 to 90 percent of posttransfusion hepatitis in the United States. In addition, it is associated with a high rate of chronicity (25 to 50 percent).

392. The answer is A (1, 2, 3). *(Blacklow, N Engl J Med 304:397–406, 1981.)* Adults are frequently infected with rotavirus. Asymptomatic rotavirus infections can occur in adult contacts. Parents of infants infected with rotavirus may have diarrhea and abdominal cramps. In addition, rotavirus is a recognized cause of travelers' diarrhea in both children and adults. Rotavirus is the most common cause of diarrhea among hospitalized children. The virus is often detected in feces for up to 8 days after the onset of disease. It is a major cause of nosocomial diarrhea among pediatric patients. In contrast to many other causes of acute enteritis, rotavirus-induced disease is frequently associated with vomiting. Infected children are most commonly between 6 and 24 months of age.

393. The answer is C (2, 4). *(Behrman, ed 12. pp 403–405.)* The prodromal features of bacterial meningitis during the first 6 months of life may be very subtle; symptoms may include lethargy and anorexia. High fever may not occur, but when present during this period, it is an extremely important sign of sepsis; urine and blood cultures and a lumbar puncture should be performed. The classic indications of meningitis—fever, stiff neck, bulging fontanelle, high-pitched cry, vomiting, and convulsions—may be absent in small infants who have the disease. In the differential diagnosis of fever in children less than 6 months of age, streptococcal pharyngitis and roseola infantum are unusual; urinary tract infections, however, must be considered carefully and are often associated with congenital anomalies involving the urinary tract.

394. The answer is E (all). *(Behrman, ed 12. pp 743–746.)* Measles is a generalized viral infection that can affect many organ systems. The disease characteristically is heralded by a severe respiratory infection that produces a harsh cough, profuse clear nasal discharge, red conjunctivae, photophobia, and high fever. A widespread, blotchy, red rash appears on the fourth or fifth day, and the symptoms worsen as the rash spreads. The rash and other symptoms abate in approximately 5 days. Koplik's spots on the buccal mucosa are pathognomonic. Complications include encephalitis, primary viral or secondary bacterial pneumonia, viral myocarditis, and otitis media. The incidence of measles in the United States has fallen dramatically as a result of the widespread use of the measles vaccine.

395. The answer is A (1, 2, 3). *(Behrman, ed 12. pp 1719–1721.)* Infection caused by *Candida albicans* ranges from a superficial mucocutaneous infection such as thrush to disseminated disease such as that occurring in newborns or patients receiving immunotherapy. Newborn infants may acquire the yeast during passage through a colonized birth canal. Final proof of invasive disease requires the demonstration of pseudohyphal forms in infected tissues. Chronic mucocutaneous candidiasis is a specific syndrome associated with immunologic defects and endocrinopathies. Amphotericin B remains the drug of choice when intravenous therapy is necessary for invasive disease.

396. The answer is E (all). *(Behrman, ed 12. pp 1710–1711.)* Allergic response to tubercle bacilli is the basis for the intracutaneous Mantoux test for tuberculosis; the test becomes positive within 2 to 10 weeks after infection. Cross-reactions to atypical mycobacteria sometimes occur and can be differentiated from positive reactions for tuberculosis by the larger intradermal reaction to the specific atypical antigen. The Mantoux test may become negative either during advanced stages of tuberculosis or briefly after immunization with live-virus vaccines (such as measles, rubella, and smallpox), administration of corticosteroids or immunosuppressive drugs, or development of a febrile illness or dehydration. Except in regions where atypical mycobacterial disease is endemic or if BCG vaccine had been given, a positive skin test in a child warrants antimicrobial therapy for at least 1 year.

397. The answer is A (1, 2, 3). *(Behrman, ed 12. pp 1223–1225.)* The x-ray that accompanies the question depicts typical features of acute osteomyelitis with periosteal new bone formation and cortical destruction. Because of the increased frequency of osteomyelitis caused by *Salmonella* and other encapsulated organisms in patients with sickle cell disease, initial therapy should include an antibiotic with known effectiveness against that organism. Many patients with sickle cell disease eventually develop functional hyposplenism and thus have a high incidence of pneumococcal bacteremia. Accordingly, prophylactic administration of polyvalent pneumococcal vaccine is recommended.

398. The answer is E (all). *(Meissner, Am J Dis Child 136:465–467, 1982.)* Lyme disease is characterized by a unique skin lesion, recurrent attacks of arthritis, and occasional involvement of the heart and central nervous system. Illness usually appears in late summer or early fall, 1 to 2 weeks after a bite by an infecting tick. Erythema chronicum migrans begins as a red macule usually on the trunk at the site of tick attachment. Nonspecific systemic signs include headache, fever, and malaise. Joint involvement generally occurs 3 to 4 weeks after onset of the rash. Cardiac disease consists primarily of rhythm disturbances. Involvement of the central nervous system is evidenced by headache and stiff neck. Treatment with penicillin does result in a faster resolution of symptoms.

399. The answer is E (all). *(Behrman, ed 12. pp 793–795.)* Poliomyelitis can be asymptomatic, producing only a brief viremia after the virus has multiplied in the intestinal tract. In both the nonparalytic and paralytic varieties, fever, sore throat, muscle pains, and aseptic meningitis with nuchal rigidity are prominent features. Complications include gastric ulcers, hypertension, bladder paralysis, and respiratory paralysis.

400. The answer is E (all). *(Behrman, ed 12. pp 651–652.)* Meningococcemia may be complicated by a variety of septic disorders, including meningitis, purulent pericarditis, endocarditis, pneumonia, otitis media, and arthritis. (Arthritis associated with meningococcemia may be mediated by an immune mechanism rather than bacterial invasion of the joint.) The potent endotoxin of the causative organism, *Neisseria meningitidis*, can induce shock, disseminated intravascular coagulation with associated hemorrhaging, and acute adrenal failure caused by localized intra-adrenal bleeding; these reactions can be collectively referred to as the Waterhouse-Friderichsen syndrome. Vaccines against *N. meningitidis* group A and C are now available, but they fail to protect young infants, who constitute a majority of the civilian population at risk. Prophylaxis with rifampin or minocycline for persons in close contact with affected individuals is recommended by many authorities.

401. The answer is A (1, 2, 3). *(Behrman, ed 12. pp 854–861.)* *Ascaris lumbri-coides* larvae travel through the intestinal wall and end up, by way of the liver, in the lungs, where they commonly produce pneumonia and peripheral eosinophilia (Loffler's syndrome); worms mature in the small intestine, where they sometimes cause obstruction. The larvae of *Toxocara canis* migrate from the intestine to all parts of the body, where granulomatous reactions may occur (visceral larva migrans). Hookworms *(Necator americanus)* can cause intestinal blood loss from mucosal laceration; cutaneous larva migrans occurs when hookworm larvae fail to enter cu-taneous blood vessels after penetrating the skin. Pinworms *(Enterobius vermicularis)* develop only in the colon, producing no internal disease other than a rare case of appendicitis. However, gravid worms crawl out of the anus at night, disturbing sleep and causing severe pruritus. Vaginitis and salpingitis may occur if the worms then enter the vagina.

402. The answer is E (all). *(Behrman ed 12. pp 410–411. Krugman, ed 7. pp 366–367, 370, 372–373.)* Colonization of a newborn infant with *Staphylococcus aureus* commonly occurs either through the skin or by way of the umbilicus, the latter leading to a purulent drainage that progresses to local redness and swelling. Although the resulting dermatitis is usually pustular, it occasionally may appear as pemphigus neonatorum, which is characterized by bulla formation, or as the "scalded skin syndrome," which features generalized erythema, tenderness, and exfoliation, especially after stroking (Nikolsky's sign). Staphylococcal neonatal mastitis is associated with a progressive enlargement of one or both breasts beyond the normal hypertrophy often noted at birth. In a newborn infant, osteomyelitis, which usually is staphylococcal, causes pseudoparalysis or point tenderness over a long bone; staphylococcal pneumonia and meningitis also can develop. Fever and other clinical signs of systemic sepsis may not be present in infants who have staphylococcal infections.

403. The answer is B (1, 3). *(Behrman, ed 12. pp 1034–1037.)* Croup involves the larynx and trachea; it usually is caused by parainfluenza or respiratory syncytial viruses. Symptoms include a low-grade fever, barking cough, and hoarse inspiratory stridor without wheezing. The pharynx may be normal or slightly red, and the lungs usually are clear. In children in severe respiratory distress, prolonged dyspnea can progress to physical exhaustion and fatal respiratory failure. Because agitation may be a sign of hypoxia, sedation should not be ordered. Hyperinflation on chest x-ray is seen in asthma, not croup.

404. The answer is E (all). *(Behrman, ed 12. pp 1028–1029.)* Most patients with otitis media do well, but temporary loss of hearing is common, secondary to fluid in the middle ear. An occasional patient will have permanent loss of hearing, secondary to damage to structures produced by the infectious process. All the complications listed in the question may occur with otitis media. Antibiotic treatment has now made these complications relatively rare, but it is important to keep them in mind in patients with otitis media so that if they occur they can be treated promptly.

405. The answer is A (1, 2, 3). *(Behrman, ed 12. pp 837, 847–850.)* Persistent, nonsuppurative diarrhea can be caused by amebas, whipworms (trichuriasis), or *Giardia lamblia*. Amebas produce an ulcerating colitis that may be very mild or extremely destructive. Amebic liver abscess should be suspected when fever, chills, leukocytosis, and right upper quadrant pain or tenderness follow diarrhea. Whipworm infection can lead to chronic irritation of the bowel wall and thus to diarrhea and rectal prolapse. Diarrhea associated with giardiasis probably occurs because of malabsorption resulting from extensive coating of intestinal mucosa by the parasite. Infestation often results from contaminated municipal or well water and is accompanied by intermittent abdominal cramps and flatulence, as well as by prolonged diarrhea. Acquired *Toxoplasma gondii* can infest any body tissue, resulting in fever, myalgia, lymphadenopathy, maculopapular rash, hepatomegaly, pneumonia, encephalitis, chorioretinitis, and myocarditis. This intracellular parasite does not ordinarily cause diarrhea and is not found in stools. Congenital toxoplasmosis may occur if a mother first acquires the parasite during pregnancy. Her infected newborn infant may demonstrate jaundice, hepatosplenomegaly, hydrocephalus or microcephaly, intracranial calcification, or chorioretinitis.

406–407. The answers are: 406-C, 407-B. *(Behrman, ed 12. pp 519–523. Rudolph, ed 17. pp 1092–1094.)* Disorders of leukocytes include (1) defective locomotion out of the bone marrow, (2) depressed chemotaxis involving cellular defects, chemotactic inhibitors, or deficiencies of chemotactic factors, and (3) inability to ingest or kill microorganisms. Sometimes several disorders are present concurrently. **Defective locomotion** results in the neutropenia characteristic of the lazy leukocyte syndrome, in which abnormal chemotaxis, otitis media, and stomatitis are also part of the clinical picture. **Depressed cellular chemotaxis** is associated with the Job-Buckley syndrome (hyperimmunoglobulin E, eczema, and recurrent staphylococcal infections), Down's syndrome, and the Chediak-Higashi syndrome (see below), among others. Inhibition of chemotaxis is seen in association with excesses of certain plasma proteins, including IgA. These excesses sometimes occur with rheumatoid arthritis, the Wiskott-Aldrich syndrome, and Hodgkin's disease. Deficiency of chemotactic factors, most of which are components of the complement system, may in association with deficient levels of complement produce recurrent, severe infections caused by encapsulated bacteria. Among the diseases associated with the **inability of leukocytes to kill ingested microorganisms** is chronic granulomatous disease. In individuals so affected, severe recurrent pneumonia and abscesses of lymph nodes and of the liver are caused by a variety of catalase-positive bacteria. These can survive ingestion by the defective leukocytes, which lack normal oxidative metabolism and cannot produce microbicidal superoxide and hydrogen peroxide. These leukocytes can be identified in the laboratory by their failure to reduce nitroblue tetrazolium (NBT tests). Chediak-Higashi syndrome is characterized by abnormally large intracytoplasmic lysosomes, visible as giant granules (Dohl bodies), which degranulate in a delayed manner after phagocytosis of pathogens. Thus, oxidative metabolism and consequent microbial killing are delayed. Neutropenia, depressed chemotaxis, and recurrent pyogenic infections are accompanying abnormalities.

408–411. The answers are: 408-B, 409-A, 410-E, 411-C. *(Behrman, ed 12. pp 504–511, 522. Rudolph, ed 17. pp 407–423.)* Many primary immunologic deficiencies may be classified as defects of T-lymphocyte function (containment of fungi, protozoa, acid-fast bacteria, and certain viruses) and B-lymphocyte function (synthesis and secretion of immunoglobulins). Among the T-cell diseases is Di George's syndrome in which defective embryologic development of the third and fourth pharyngeal pouches results in hypoplasia of both thymus and parathyroid glands.

Primary B-cell diseases include panhypogammaglobulinemia (Bruton's disease), an X-linked deficiency of all three major classes of immunoglobulins, as well as other selective deficiencies of the immunoglobulins or their subgroups.

Combined T- and B-cell diseases include the X-linked recessive Wiskott-Aldrich syndrome of mild T-cell dysfunction, diminished serum IgM, marked elevation of IgA and IgE, eczema, recurrent middle ear infections, lymphopenia, and thrombocytopenia.

Patients with the catastrophic combined T- and B-cell disease known as combined immunodeficiency disease (Swiss-type lymphopenic agammaglobulinemia) have deficient T and B cells. Consequently, there are both marked lymphopenia and agammaglobulinemia, as well as hypoplasia of the thymus. Chronic diarrhea, rashes, recurrent serious bacterial, fungal, or viral infections, wasting, and early death are characteristic. Other T- and B-cell deficiencies include ataxia-telangiectasia and chronic mucocutaneous candidiasis.

Job-Buckley syndrome is a disorder of phagocyte chemotaxis associated with hypergammaglobulin E, eczema, and recurrent severe staphylococcal infections.

Hematologic and Neoplastic Diseases

DIRECTIONS: Each question below contains five suggested responses. Select the **one best** response to each question.

412. Thrombocytopenia in the newborn is associated with all the following EXCEPT

(A) congenital cytomegalovirus infection
(B) perinatal aspiration syndrome
(C) maternal idiopathic thrombocytopenic purpura (ITP)
(D) maternal ingestion of aspirin
(E) absence of radii in the infant

413. The most common cause of death in children who have homozygous beta-thalassemia is

(A) hepatic insufficiency
(B) diabetes mellitus
(C) cardiac arrhythmias and congestive heart failure
(D overwhelming bacterial sepsis
(E) hypoadrenalism

414. A 15-month-old boy presents with recurrent furuncles for a duration of 3 months. He has not had any serious infection that requires hospitalization. Physical examination reveals a few palpable cervical and inguinal lymph nodes and two furuncles at the perirectal region. His white count is 5100/mm^3 with a differential of 6 percent polymorphonuclear neutrophils, 3 percent monocytes, and 1 percent eosinophils and 90 percent lymphocytes. The LEAST likely diagnosis is

(A) cyclic neutropenia
(B) benign childhood neutropenia
(C) Kostman's syndrome
(D) dilantin therapy
(E) acute leukemia

415. The spleen indisputably shortens red blood cell survival in which of the following conditions?

(A) Pyruvate kinase deficiency
(B) Hexokinase deficiency
(C) Glucose-6-phosphate dehydrogenase deficiency
(D) Hereditary spherocytosis
(E) Acquired idiopathic hemolytic anemia

416. A 6-month-old infant presents with failure to thrive, psychomotor deterioration, and hepatosplenomegaly. Wright-Giemsa staining of a bone marrow aspirate shows large numbers of cells, as illustrated below. These findings are associated most closely with

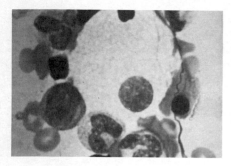

(A) histiocytosis X
(B) Gaucher's disease
(C) Niemann-Pick disease
(D) Hurler's syndrome
(E) myelogenous leukemia

417. A 10-year-old boy is admitted to the hospital because of bleeding. Pertinent laboratory findings include a platelet count of 50,000/mm^3, prothrombin time (PT) of 15 s (control 11.5 s), activated partial thromboplastin time (aPTT) of 51 s (control 36 s), thrombin time (TT) of 13.7 s (control 10.5 s), and factor VIII level 14 percent (normal 38–178 percent). The most likely cause of his bleeding is

(A) idiopathic thrombocytopenic purpura (ITP)
(B) hemophilia A
(C) disseminated intravascular coagulation (DIC)
(D) liver disease
(E) vitamin K deficiency

418. A 6-year-old girl is hospitalized because of pallor and fatigue of a few weeks' duration. When she was 18 months of age, she had iron deficiency anemia that responded to oral iron and blood transfusion therapy; at that time a stool guaiac of 3+ was attributed to excessive milk intake. When she was 4 years of age, her anemia recurred; treatment with intramuscular iron was effective. Except for her pallor, physical examination is unremarkable. Laboratory results are hemoglobin, 5 g per 100 ml; reticulocytes, 3 percent; and microcytic, hypochromic erythrocytes in the peripheral blood smear. Neither the child nor her parents have been aware of her having gastrointestinal symptoms or blood in the stools.

The cause of this child's anemia would best be established by

(A) screening for sickle cell hemoglobin
(B) testing for serum iron and total iron-binding capacity
(C) a hemolytic workup
(D) a barium study of the gastrointestinal tract
(E) a red blood cell survival test (^{51}chromium labeling)

419. All the following statements are associated with children and adolescents with sickle cell anemia EXCEPT that

(A) height and weight are reduced as compared with national health statistical norms
(B) bone age is delayed
(C) there is delayed sexual maturation
(D) the plasma concentrations of pituitary gonadotropin do not rise during puberty
(E) the incidence of cholelithiasis increases during adolescence

420. The following statements concerning side effects of antineoplastic agents are true EXCEPT that

(A) vincristine can cause peripheral neuropathy
(B) prednisone can cause alopecia
(C) methotrexate can cause mucositis
(D) 6-mercaptopurine can cause hepatic dysfunction
(E) doxorubicin (Adriamycin) can cause cardiomyopathy

421. Premature infants 3 to 6 months of age and older are more prone to develop significant anemia than are comparably aged full-term infants. This late anemia of prematurity is most likely to be the consequence of

(A) a lack of erythropoietin synthesis
(B) a decreased oxygen requirement and an increased oxygen unloading capacity
(C) decreased red blood cell survival
(D) rapid growth and diminished iron reserves
(E) poor utilization of available iron in food

422. Neuroblastoma can be associated with all the following statements EXCEPT that

(A) approximately 50 percent of neuroblastomas occur during the first 2 years of life
(B) heterochromia iridis and Horner's syndrome may be manifestations of cervical neuroblastoma
(C) metastases are uncommon at the time of diagnosis
(D) serial measurements of urinary catecholamines are useful in predicting the progression of neuroblastoma
(E) spontaneous regression is known to occur in neuroblastoma

423. All the following statements regarding Hodgkin's disease are true EXCEPT that

(A) Hodgkin's disease is very rare before the age of 5 years, but there is a peak of incidence at 15 to 34 years
(B) fever and night sweats can be presenting symptoms of Hodgkin's disease
(C) eosinophilia can be an associated finding
(D) in most patients with Hodgkin's disease, the initial mode of spread occurs via lymphatic channels to contiguous lymph nodes
(E) staging laparotomy is mandatory in every patient with Hodgkin's disease

424. All the following statements regarding Burkitt's lymphoma are true EXCEPT that

—(A) Burkitt's lymphoma is the most common form of lymphoma in children in the United States
(B) Burkitt's lymphoma in Africa is almost always associated with Epstein-Barr virus (EBV)
(C) translocation of chromatin from chromosome 8 to 14 t(8;14) is a common cytogenetic abnormality
(D) Burkitt's lymphoma is a form of B-cell lymphoma
(E) with modern aggressive combination chemotherapy over 50 percent of patients with Burkitt's lymphoma can be expected to have prolonged survival

425. All the following statements regarding medulloblastoma are true EXCEPT that

(A) the incidence of medulloblastoma is increased in individuals with the basal cell nevus syndrome
⤙ (B) the most common location of medulloblastoma in children is in one of the cerebellar hemispheres
(C) medulloblastoma frequently metastasizes along the pathway of the cerebrospinal fluid (CSF)
(D) medulloblastoma is usually a radiosensitive tumor
(E) the level of polyamines in the CSF of many patients with medulloblastoma is elevated

426. All the following statements about the treatment of childhood acute lymphoblastic leukemia are true EXCEPT that

(A) the use of vincristine and prednisone can produce remission in 80 to 90 percent of patients
(B) patients who fail to achieve remission after 4 weeks of induction therapy have a poor prognosis
(C) effective presymptomatic treatment of the central nervous system after remission induction has resulted in a decrease in the incidence of meningeal relapse from over 50 percent to less than 10 percent
(D) patients who relapse in the bone marrow while on treatment can still achieve remission in 90 percent of cases but the remission is usually short lived
—(E) approximately 50 percent of patients relapse after discontinuation of therapy

427. The polymorphonuclear neutrophil shown in the illustration below is
most likely to be associated with

(A) malignancy
(B) iron deficiency
— (C) folic acid deficiency
(D) Döhle's inclusion bodies
(E) the Pelger-Huët nuclear anomaly

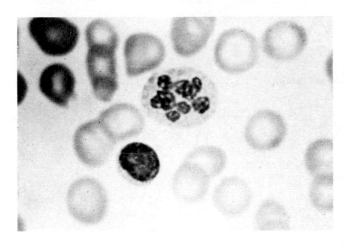

DIRECTIONS: Each question below contains four suggested responses of which **one or more** is correct. Select

A	if	**1, 2, and 3**	are correct
B	if	**1 and 3**	are correct
C	if	**2 and 4**	are correct
D	if	**4**	is correct
E	if	**1, 2, 3, and 4**	are correct

428. Correct statements about osteosarcoma include which of the following?

— (1) Osteosarcoma is rare in preschool children, but its incidence sharply rises during adolescence

— (2) About 50 percent of osteosarcomas occur in the area of the knee (distal femur or proximal tibia or fibula)

— (3) The most common sites of metastasis are the lungs and pleura

(4) The role of current adjuvant chemotherapy after ablative surgery in improving cure rate is well defined

429. Poor prognostic signs in children who have acute lymphocytic leukemia include which of the following?

—(1) Age below 2 years or above 10 years

—(2) Median white blood cell count at diagnosis of 20,000/mm^3 or more

— (3) Presence of mediastinal mass

— (4) Early central nervous system leukemia

430. A 2-year-old child in shock has fulminant meningococcemia; petechiae are noted, and oozing from puncture sites has been observed. The child's peripheral blood smear, presented below, shows fragmented red blood cells and few platelets. Clotting studies are likely to show

— (1) decreased levels of factors V and VIII
— (2) a decreased prothrombin level
— (3) a decreased fibrinogen level
— (4) the presence of fibrin split products

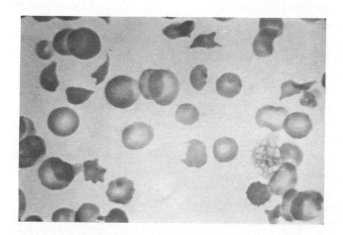

431. Hypochromic anemia is likely to be associated with which of the following disorders?

— (1) Iron deficiency
— (2) Anemia owing to lead intoxication
— (3) Thalassemia
— (4) Pyridoxine-responsive anemia

432. Splenectomy for a 2-year-old child has been recommended. In regard to the child's risk of developing an overwhelming infection after surgery it is true that

— (1) institution of high-dose penicillin therapy for febrile illnesses can reduce the risk
— (2) salvaging of at least part of the spleen, if possible, can reduce the risk
— (3) immunization with pneumococcal polysaccharide vaccine can reduce the risk
— (4) the risk is higher in this child than in a splenectomized 4-year-old child

433. The overall prevalence of iron deficiency anemia in American children between the ages of 6 months and 2 years has remained stable during the last 3 decades despite the increasing availability of iron-fortified foods. True statements regarding preventive measures against iron deficiency anemia include which of the following?

(1) Breast milk is a better source of iron than cow's milk

(2) Cow's milk is a better source of iron than commercial formulas

(3) Iron supplementation for premature infants should begin at 2 months of age

(4) The best commercial cereals are those containing sodium iron pyrophosphate

434. Incidental factors affecting hemoglobin concentration and hematocrit values in a normal newborn infant include

(1) the site of blood sampling
(2) previous fetomaternal blood exchange
(3) the length of time between birth and blood sampling
(4) the manner in which the umbilical cord is clamped at the time of delivery

435. Because of fetal distress, labor is induced at 41 weeks gestation in a 40-year-old diabetic mother who has moderate toxemia of pregnancy. Induction of labor leads to the spontaneous delivery of an infant who on examination is small for gestational age, looks plethoric, and is in mild respiratory distress. Signs of Down's syndrome also are present. Laboratory data include a venous hemoglobin concentration of 26 g per 100 ml and a venous hematocrit of 75%.

The polycythemia in this newborn may be attributable to

(1) maternal diabetes
(2) placental insufficiency
(3) maternal-fetal transfusion
(4) Down's syndrome

436. Assay of serum ferritin is a new tool in evaluating iron nutrition. Its advantages over the traditional measurements of hemoglobin, hematocrit, and serum transferrin saturation include which of the following?

(1) It allows evaluation of iron status within the normal range as well as in deficiency and excess

(2) Return of serum ferritin to normal levels reflects the effect of iron supplementation more reliably than do such returns of hematocrit and transferrin saturation

(3) In anemia caused by infection or chronic disease, consistently elevated values of serum ferritin are a more reliable indicator of iron status than are values of transferrin saturation

(4) Serum ferritin is a better estimate of a mobile pool of iron than transferrin saturation

437. A preterm black male infant was found to be jaundiced 12 hours after birth. At 36 hours of age, his serum bilirubin was 18 mg/dl, hemoglobin concentration was 12.5 g/dl, and reticulocyte count 9 percent. Many nucleated red cells and some spherocytes were seen in the peripheral blood smear. The differential diagnosis should include

(1) glucose-6-phosphate dehydrogenase (G-6-PD) deficiency

(2) hereditary spherocytosis

(3) ABO incompatibility

(4) Rh incompatibility

DIRECTIONS: Each group of questions below consists of lettered headings followed by a set of numbered items. For each numbered item select the **one** lettered heading with which it is **most** closely associated. Each lettered heading may be used **once, more than once, or not at all.**

Questions 438–442

For each disorder listed below, select the peripheral blood smear with which it is most likely to be associated.

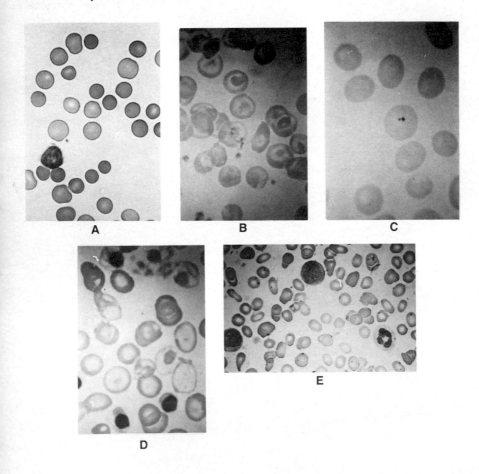

438. Howell-Jolly bodies in a splenectomized child

439. Basophilic stippling in a child who has lead intoxication

440. Thalassemia major

441. Hereditary spherocytosis

442. Hemoglobin C disease

Questions 443–445

For each type of childhood leukemia listed below, choose the bone marrow photomicrograph with which it is most likely to be associated.

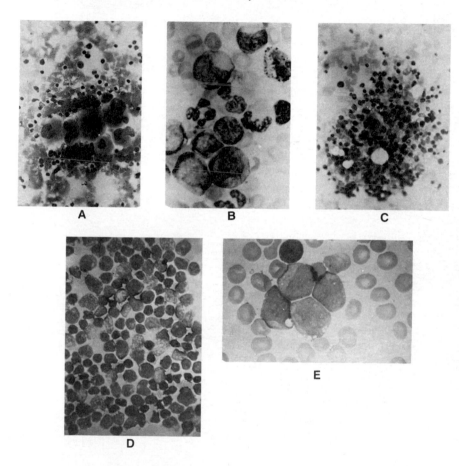

A   B   C

D

E

443. Acute lymphoblastic leukemia (ALL)

444. Acute myeloblastic leukemia (AML)

445. Chronic granulocytic leukemia (CGL)

Questions 446–450

Match the following chemotherapeutic agents with their corresponding
mechanisms of action (as supported by
cell kinetic studies).

446. Cyclophosphamide

447. 6-Mercaptopurine

448. Methotrexate

449. Cytosine arabinoside

450. Vincristine

(A) Impairs DNA synthesis by
competitive inhibition of DNA
polymerase
(B) Damages the microtubules in
the mitotic spindle
(C) Alkylates purine bases in the
DNA chain, leading to inhibition of DNA synthesis
(D) Binds to dehydrofolate reductase to prevent pyrimidine
synthesis
(E) Blocks purine synthesis by inhibiting key enzymatic reactions

Hematologic and Neoplastic Diseases

Answers

412.   The answer is D. *(Cines, N Engl J Med 306:826, 1982. Oski, ed 3. p 184.)* Thrombocytopenia and hemolytic anemia are common manifestations of the TORCH (toxoplasmosis, rubella, cytomegalovirus, and herpes simplex) infections as well as congenital syphilis. Both increased platelet destruction and impaired production of platelets may be the mechanism involved. Aspiration of amniotic fluid can lead to thrombocytopenia, probably because of amniotic fluid-induced platelet aggregation in the pulmonary capillary bed. Some mothers who have had ITP and who have high levels of antiplatelet antibody in the maternal plasma can give birth to thrombocytopenic infants owing to transplacental crossing of antiplatelet IgG antibody. The syndrome of congenital amegakaryocytic thrombocytopenia and bilateral absence of the radii is a well-known entity. Maternal ingestion of aspirin can lead to bleeding in the newborn, not as a result of thrombocytopenia but as a consequence of transient impairment of the infant's platelet aggregation.

413.   The answer is C. *(Nathan, ed 2. pp 726–799.)* Homozygous beta-thalassemia, or Cooley's anemia, is a severe inherited anemia caused by decreased synthesis of beta globin chains. Almost every patient requires frequent transfusion therapy. Each 250 ml unit of packed red blood cells contains approximately 250 mg of iron; the usual requirement of 2 units every 3 or 4 weeks will result in an excess accumulation of 50 g of iron in 10 years. (The total body iron in a normal adult is 4 to 5 g.) These patients also have increased iron absorption owing to excess erythropoiesis and some hypoxia owing to anemia. This excess iron can damage liver, spleen, pancreas, and almost any other organ, but the worst effect is on the heart. Acute pericarditis is a rather benign complication that has its onset at about 11 years of age; it afflicted 19 of 46 patients in one series. However, cardiac arrhythmias and congestive heart failure were the leading causes of death in this series (24 to 25 patients). The average age of onset was 16 years; 14 patients died within 3 months of onset of this complication, and only 7 patients lived more than 1 year after the onset of heart failure. Autopsy findings showed severe myocardial hemosiderosis. More effective chelation therapy may postpone this inevitable complication.

414.   The answer is C. *(Nathan, ed 2. pp 838–845.)* Neutropenia in children can arise from disorders of proliferation of committed stem cells (such as cyclic neutropenia) or from disorders of proliferation of committed myeloid stem cells (such as benign neutropenia and Kostman's syndrome). Neutropenia can also be associated with abnormalities of the T and B lymphocytes, phenotypic abnormalities (such as Shwachman-Diamond syndrome and cartilage-hair hypoplasia), bone marrow replacement (such as leukemia and lymphoma), vitamin B_{12} or folate deficiency, bone marrow suppression by drugs (such as sulfonamides and anticonvulsants), certain infections, immune-mediated destruction of neutrophils, and hypersplenism. In this patient, the absence of a past history of serious infection makes Kostman's syndrome the least likely diagnosis because Kostman's syndrome, usually an autosomal recessive disorder, is associated with chronic severe neutropenia and severe and often lethal pyogenic infections of the skin and respiratory tract, usually beginning during the first month of life. The outcome is usually fatal in early life.

415. The answer is D. *(Lux, Pediatr Clin North Am 27:463–486, 1980. Sullivan, Pediatr Ann 9:38–42, 1980.)* During its usual life span of 120 days, the red cell not only must maintain an adequate energy supply through utilization of glucose, but it also must keep a structural integrity and deformability to be able to negotiate its passage through small capillaries (2 to 3 μ) and the mechanically and metabolically stressful environment of the spleen. In the last few years, new data about red cell structural proteins and membrane skeleton (spectrin, actin, and ankyrin) suggest the existence of a qualitative defect that renders hereditary spherocytic red cells unstable and easily fragmented. The sequence of changes that ends with red cell death begins with loss of membrane fragments, which causes a decreased surface area/volume ratio (spherocytosis), with decreased cellular deformability. This leads to splenic entrapment and red cell death. The congested, acidic, hypoglycemic environment of the splenic cords accelerates spherocyte formation in hereditary spherocytosis (HS) more than in other conditions. Because it abolishes the hemolytic process, splenectomy is almost curative in HS. The red cells take on a more uniform morphology after splenectomy. Although splenectomy may be of marginal benefit in pyruvate kinase deficiency and hexokinase deficiency, it is of no benefit in glucose-6-phosphate dehydrogenase deficiency and acquired idiopathic hemolytic anemia.

416. The answer is C. *(Williams, ed 2. pp 1151–1152.)* The clinical history and the presence of foam cells in the bone marrow of the infant described in the question are typical of Niemann-Pick disease (sphingomyelin lipidosis). A deficiency of the lysosomal enzyme sphingomyelinase in several tissues causes the accumulation of sphingomyelin, which is ingested by reticuloendothelial cells. The resulting rounded or oval cells (foam cells) have an eccentric nucleus with prominent nucleoli; however, the distinguishing characteristic is the appearance of small, glittering droplets in the cytoplasm. These abnormal cells can be found in the bone marrow, liver, spleen, lymph nodes, thymus, brain, and many other organs. The foam cells of Gaucher's disease typically look different; the cytoplasm of these Gaucher's cells appears to be stuffed with many long, wavy fibrils of variable length, giving the appearance of wrinkled tissue paper.

417. The answer is C. *(Nathan, ed 2. pp 1189–1235.)* The prolongation of PT, aPTT, and TT excludes the diagnosis of ITP. PT tests principally for factors I, II, V, VII, and X and is not prolonged in hemophilia A (factor VIII deficiency). In liver disease PT, aPTT, and TT are all prolonged, but the level of factor VIII, which is not synthesized in the liver, is normal and the platelet count is usually normal unless there is associated hypersplenism. In vitamin K deficiency there is a decrease in the production of factors II, VII, IX, and X, and PT and aPTT are prolonged. However, the thrombin time, which tests for conversion of fibrinogen to fibrin, should be normal and the platelet count should also be normal. In DIC, there is consumption of fibrinogen, factors II, V, and VIII, and platelets. Therefore, there is prolongation of PT, aPTT, and TT and decrease in factor VIII level and platelet count. In addition, the titer of fibrin split production is usually increased.

418. The answer is D. *(Nathan, ed 2. pp 315–321.)* Intestinal blood loss is frequently a contributing factor in the pathogenesis of iron deficiency anemia. This blood loss almost always ceases once iron replacement treatment is started and intake of cow's milk is reduced. Blood loss also can occur from anatomic lesions, such as Meckel's diverticula, intestinal duplications, hemorrhagic telangiectasia, or bleeding ulcers; unfortunately, these are easily overlooked in a child because of their uncommon occurrence and paucity of symptoms. Blood loss caused by these lesions must be suspected in anemic children older than 2 years of age or whose intestinal blood loss or anemia persists or recurs after iron treatment.

Two errors were made in the management of the patient presented in the question. First, the presence of occult blood in the stool should have been tested after the initiation of iron treatment at 18 months of age. Second and more significant, when the child was 4 years of age and iron deficiency anemia recurred, an immediate search for occult blood loss should have begun. A hemolytic anemia is not suggested by the data presented, and it certainly would not have responded to iron therapy.

419. The answer is D. *(Karayalcin, Am J Dis Child 133:306, 1979. Luban, Am J Pediatr Hematol/Oncol 4:61–65, 1982.)* In a longitudinal study of children with sickle cell anemia, their height and weight were found to be significantly reduced and their bone ages were significantly retarded. The Tanner staging was appropriate for bone age rather than chronological age, suggesting delayed maturation. However, the pituitary gonadotropins were found to be increased during puberty, and the thyroid and adrenal function tests were also normal, suggesting an intact pituitary-hypothalamic axis. In one series, cholelithiasis was found in 8 of 47 patients aged 2 to 18 years; 6 out of the 8 patients with cholelithiasis were aged 10 years or older.

420. The answer is B. *(Altman, ed 2. pp 59–95.)* The main toxicities of vincristine include neuropathy (sensory, motor, autonomic, or cranial nerve), constipation, jaw pain, alopecia, and inappropriate antidiuretic hormone secretion. The major side effects of prednisone include cushingoid facies, truncal obesity, salt and water retention, hypertension, increased susceptibility to infection, gastric irritation, and osteoporosis. The toxicity of methotrexate is dependent on the dose, schedule, and route of administration. The major toxicities include gastrointestinal mucositis, bone marrow suppression, skin erythema, and hepatic dysfunction. 6-Mercaptopurine can cause nausea, vomiting, marrow suppression, and hepatic dysfunction. Doxorubicin (Adriamycin) can lead to alopecia, nausea, vomiting, stomatitis, tissue necrosis (if drug extravasates), and bone marrow suppression. The dose-limiting factor is cardiotoxicity, and the risk of cardiotoxicity increases at cumulative doses of doxorubicin above 550 mg/M^2.

421. The answer is D. *(Forbes, pp 215–216. Nathan, ed 2. pp 309–311.)* It is generally accepted that late anemia of prematurity stems from nutritional deficiencies (largely iron deficiency) caused by rapid growth and early depletion of already poor reserves. Full-term and premature newborns begin life with standard iron reserves of approximately 70 mg/kg body weight. In contrast to full-term infants whose birth weights double by 5 months of age and triple by 1 year of age, premature infants may triple their birth weights by 6 months of age. Early physiologic anemia of newborn infants, which is most evident between 6 and 12 weeks after birth, results from decreased red blood cell survival, decreased oxygen requirements, increased oxygen unloading capacity, and an absence of erythropoietin synthesis. These factors are all common in newborns but are somewhat more pronounced in premature infants. This is why iron supplementation is recommended for premature infants at 2 months of age.

422. The answer is C. *(Levine, pp 663–682.)* Neuroblastoma is a malignancy seen predominantly in the young, reflecting the congenital nature of its origin. About half of the neuroblastomas occur during the first 2 years of life. Neuroblastoma can arise anywhere along the course of the sympathetic nervous system. Involvement of the cervical or upper thoracic sympathetic nervous system can manifest with Horner's syndrome or heterochromia iridis. Two thirds of patients, when first seen, have metastases, especially to liver, bones, bone marrow, skin, and lymph nodes. Approximately three fourths of all tumors secrete catecholamines (vanillyl mandelic acid and homovanillic acid). Serial measurements of the urinary catecholamines aid a correct prognosis. The 2-year survival rate is significantly better in patients in whom the urinary catecholamine levels normalize as compared with patients in whom the levels fail to normalize or increase progressively.

423. The answer is E. *(Altman, ed 2. pp 297–329.)* In underdeveloped countries the peak incidence of Hodgkin's disease is under 10 years of age; however, in the developed countries the peak incidence occurs in late adolescence and young adulthood. There is a late peak after the age of 50. Systemic symptoms of Hodgkin's disease include fever, night sweats, malaise, weight loss, and pruritus. However, in the Ann Arbor Staging System only fever, night sweats, and weight loss are considered significant systemic symptoms that have prognostic importance. Neutrophilia occurs in about 50 percent of patients and eosinophilia in 15 to 20 percent of patients. In most instances the initial mode of spread of Hodgkin's disease is predictable involvement of contiguous lymphoid tissue. The objective of surgical staging is to determine whether there is occult intraabdominal disease in patients who clinically have only apparent supradiaphragmatic involvement. The information provided by staging laparotomy is important if radiation therapy is the only modality of treatment contemplated. In patients who have obvious intraabdominal disease by noninvasive studies (such as CAT scan or lymphangiogram) or obvious metastases outside the lymphatic system (e.g., bone marrow), combination chemotherapy with or without radiation therapy is generally recommended and staging laparotomy is then not required.

424. The answer is A. *(Levine, pp 473–574.)* Burkitt's lymphoma, a form of B-cell lymphoma, although common in equatorial Africa (100 per million children), is a very rare form of lymphoma in children in the United States (1 to 2 per million children). EBV is almost always associated with the African variety of Burkitt's lymphoma but is uncommonly connected with Burkitt's lymphoma diagnosed in the United States. t(8;14) is a very common cytogenetic abnormality in Burkitt's lymphoma. Prior to the modern combination chemotherapy era, very few children with Burkitt's lymphoma achieved prolonged survival. Current intensive chemotherapy with cyclophosphamide, doxorubicin, vincristine, prednisone, and methotrexate can produce prolonged survival in over 50 percent of patients.

425. The answer is B. *(Altman, ed 2. pp 347–767.)* Primary brain tumors, such as medulloblastoma, occur with increased frequency in patients with ataxia telangiectasia, basal cell nevus syndrome, hereditary neurocutaneous disorders, and familial glioma polyposis syndrome. In children, medulloblastoma is usually a midline tumor most probably arising from the posterior medullary velum; in older adolescents and adults there is an increased incidence of medulloblastoma arising from the cerebellar hemispheres. Medulloblastomas usually spread along the pathway of the CSF and can seed many parts of the brain and spinal cord. Rarely, medulloblastoma can spread outside the nervous system to bone, bone marrow, lymph nodes, or abdominal cavity (via a ventriculoperitoneal shunt). The standard treatment is surgical resection followed by irradiation of the craniospinal axis. Trials of adjuvant chemotherapy have shown promise, and the role of chemotherapy will be better defined in the near future. The level of CSF polyamines is elevated in many patients with medulloblastoma and can be used to monitor progress of disease or to detect early recurrence.

426. The answer is E. *(Altman, ed 2. pp 239–296.)* Vincristine and prednisone are the standard drugs used in remission induction for childhood acute lymphoblastic leukemia. L-Asparaginase is usually added either during induction or during consolidation therapy. Patients who fail to achieve either complete remission on day

28, or partial remission on day 14, have a poor prognosis, even if they attain remission with subsequent therapy. The introduction of cranial irradiation with intrathecal methotrexate or intravenous intermediate dose methotrexate and intrathecal methotrexate in certain patients has reduced the incidence of meningeal relapse from over 50 percent to under 10 percent. Bone marrow relapse while on therapy signifies a very poor prognosis, although remission is still usually achievable with chemotherapy. Recent studies suggest that bone marrow transplantation may improve the survival of some of these patients. The optimal duration of therapy is still not clearly defined. Most patients have their therapy discontinued after 2 to 3 years of continuous remission. About 15 to 25 percent of patients relapse after cessation of therapy, usually within the first year.

427. The answer is C. *(Lindenbaum, Br J Haematol 44:511–513, 1980. Nathan, ed 2. pp 349–352.)* The finding of hypersegmented neutrophils in the peripheral blood is one of the most useful laboratory aids in making an early diagnosis of folate deficiency. In adults put on a folate-deficient diet, serum folate levels become low in 3 weeks, and hypersegmented neutrophils appear in the bone marrow in 5 weeks and in the peripheral blood in 7 weeks. It is only after 17 or 19 weeks that megaloblastic anemia develops. In a recent retrospective study of 357 patients with megaloblastic anemia, in 351 patients, the peripheral blood smear was found to have at least one hypersegmented neutrophil with six or more lobes per 100 cells. In contrast, only 1 of the 50 controls had a single six-lobed neutrophil. The Pelger-Huët anomaly is an inherited disorder in which neutrophils have no more than two lobes. Neutrophils in severe bacterial infections have toxic granulation, Döhle's inclusion bodies, and cytoplasmic vacuoles.

428. The answer is A (1, 2, 3). *(Levine, pp 575–602.)* Osteosarcoma is a tumor primarily of the 10- to 20-year-old age group, suggesting a correlation between the occurrence of the tumor and the rate of bone growth. It most frequently affects the metaphyses of long bones, especially the distal femur and proximal tibia or fibula. Although lungs and pleura are the most common sites of metastases, the tumor can also spread to other bones, lymph nodes, pericardium, kidneys, brain, and adrenal glands. There are controversies regarding the beneficial role of adjuvant chemotherapy after ablative surgery. Although many trials on chemotherapy have been performed, they were mostly nonrandomized studies, and the ultimate disease-free survival has been about 45 to 50 percent. Investigators at the Mayo Clinic have reported in a small randomized study that an actuarial 2-year relapse-free survival of 52 percent was observed with or without adjuvant chemotherapy. A multicentered randomized study is now in progress.

429. The answer is E (all). *(Altman, ed 2. pp 253–256. Mauer, Blood 56:1–10, 1980.)* Age less than 2 years or more than 10 years, the presence at diagnosis of central nervous system leukemia or a white blood cell count of 20,000/mm³ or higher, and the appearance of a mediastinal mass all indicate a poor prognosis for children who have acute lymphocytic leukemia. Most of the children having these poor prognostic signs have the thymic (T cell) variety of the disease. These children, usually older boys, possess surface antigens specific for thymocytes. In addition to the conventionally employed regimen of prednisone and vincristine, other chemotherapeutic agents, such as daunorubicin or L-asparaginase, should be administered. Children with T-cell acute lymphocytic leukemia run a greater risk of bleeding and infection during the first 4 weeks of remission induction therapy. Only 20 percent of these patients with poor prognostic features can be expected to achieve long-term disease-free survival, and once they relapse, which is very often in the first few months, virtually none of them go into remission despite aggressive chemotherapy.

430. The answer is E (all). *(Nathan, ed 2. pp 1223–1228.)* The clinical history and blood-smear findings presented in the question are typical of disseminated intravascular coagulation. The disorder, which can be triggered by endotoxin shock, results ultimately in the initiation of the intrinsic clotting mechanism and the generation of thrombin. Fibrin deposited in the microcirculatory system can lead to tissue ischemia and necrosis, further capillary damage, release of thromboplastic substances, and increased thrombin generation. Simultaneous activation of the fibrinolytic system produces increased amounts of fibrin split products, which inhibit thrombin activity. Of utmost importance in the treatment of children who have disseminated intravascular coagulation is the management of the condition that precipitated the disorder.

431. The answer is E (all). *(Nathan, ed 2. pp 329–332.)* Red blood cells emerging from the bone marrow with decreased amounts of hemoglobin first become smaller (microcytic) in order to sustain an adequate mean corpuscular hemoglobin concentration and only later become hypochromic and show increased central pallor on peripheral-smear examination. The impairment could be in the synthesis of globin or heme. In thalassemia, there is a quantitative decrease in globin-chain synthesis owing to a genetic disorder. In iron deficiency, synthesis of heme is impaired owing to lack of iron; and lead can block incompletely many enzymatic steps in heme manufacture. In pyridoxine-responsive anemia, the exact mechanism causing hypochromicity is unknown, but the impairments resemble those of lead poisoning and result in poor utilization of adequate iron stores situated in the normoblasts.

432. The answer is E (all). *(Gellis, pp 276–278.)* The immune functions of the spleen, other than the filtration and phagocytosis of bacteria in the reticuloendothelial system, are not completely known. After splenectomy, the serum level of immunoglobulin M falls and opsonization of encapsulated organisms like *Streptococcus (Diplococcus) pneumoniae* becomes defective. These factors may contribute to the development of overwhelming pneumococcal infections in splenectomized children, especially those who are less than 4 years of age, who have a severe hematologic disease, or who require chemotherapy for lymphoma. A recent follow-up evaluation of 71 splenectomized or autosplenectomized patients who were immunized with pneumococcal polysaccharide vaccine revealed that this vaccine is effective in preventing pneumococcal sepsis. Although the use of prophylactic penicillin in splenectomized children has been recommended, it is not known for how many years prophylaxis should be continued or whether it can prevent sepsis caused by gram-negative organisms. An aggressive approach to febrile illness in children should be undertaken, including institution of high-dose penicillin therapy before blood culture results are available.

433. The answer is B (1, 3) *(AAP-CN, Pediatrics 58:765–768, 1976. Dallman, p 6.)* The Committee of Nutrition of the American Academy of Pediatrics states that iron supplementation from one or two sources, such as the newer iron-fortified cereals (that do not contain the poorly absorbed iron pyrophosphate) or iron-containing drops, should begin at 4 months of age for term infants and 2 months for premature infants. Breast-feeding is preferred, and iron-fortified formulas and other heat-treated milk products are better than cow's milk as substitutes for human breast milk during the first 6 to 12 months of an infant's life. After the age of 6 months, infants receiving cow's milk should have their daily milk intake limited to 750 ml and should begin eating iron-rich solid foods. Excessive milk ingestion increases occult blood loss in the gastrointestinal tract and thus contributes to iron deficiency anemia. Unless milk drinking is discouraged and better methods of iron supplementation for infants are adopted, iron deficiency will remain all too common. It has recently been shown by using an external tagging method ($^{59}FeSO_4$) that breast-fed infants absorb 49 percent of the iron in the breast milk in contrast with infants fed cow's milk or unfortified cow's milk formula who absorbed only 10 to 12 percent of the available iron. Assessment of iron nutrition by serum ferritin measurements indicates that routine iron supplementation may not be necessary in term infants who continue to be breast-fed.

434. The answer is E (all). *(Nathan, ed 2. pp 27–31.)* Capillary blood samples from a heel prick have hemoglobin values 10 percent higher than venous samples. This error can be minimized by warming the area, eliciting a brisk blood flow, and discarding the initial drops. Within the first few hours after birth, plasma volume decreases and hemoglobin concentration increases (from 15 to 25 percent). The placental vessels at birth contain 75 to 125 ml of blood, about a quarter of which normally gets into a newborn infant within 15 seconds of birth. Cord-related factors can make a difference of 40 percent of neonatal blood volume; for example, because the umbilical arteries constrict shortly after birth, whereas the vein remains dilated, delayed cord clamping was associated in one study with an average red blood cell mass of 49 ml/kg at 72 hours as compared with 31 ml/kg in infants with immediate cord clamping. Fetomaternal transfusion in the last phases of pregnancy and labor can lead to anemia in the newborn; conversely, maternal-fetal transfusion can result in plethora.

435. The answer is E (all). *(Nathan, ed 2. pp 1509–1510.)* Polycythemia (hemoglobin, > 22 g per 100 ml; hematocrit, > 65%) in an infant during the first week of life can lead to several undesirable complications. Although the etiology may be obscure, placental insufficiency leading to intrauterine hypoxia seems to play a central role in the majority of the conditions associated with plethora. Maternal diabetes, another common cause, may be related to placental dysfunction. In infants who have Down's syndrome, evidence of a myeloproliferative disorder is not uncommon; it can affect in the neonatal period any of the formed blood elements and very often is associated with myeloid hyperplasia that can be confused with congenital leukemia.

436. The answer is A (1, 2, 3). *(Nathan, ed 2. pp 217–218.)* Serum ferritin concentration is a very sensitive reflection of iron stores from birth to adult life. Its assay requires less than 0.1 ml of serum, and because samples can be stored for several months, it is a useful tool in nutritional surveys. In the natural sequence of stages in iron deficiency, depletion of *iron stores,* as manifested by a fall in serum ferritin concentration, is the first readily detectable event. This is then followed by a fall in serum transferrin saturation (which represents the *mobile iron pool*). Only when transferrin saturation drops below 15 percent does the marrow feel the pinch of iron deficiency. Anemia is a late nonspecific manifestation of iron deficiency; in fact, iron deficiency, as reflected first by decreased ferritin levels and then by transferrin saturation, may exist for several weeks before there are clinical manifestations of anemia. Infection and chronic disease may cause transferrin synthesis but not serum ferritin concentration to drop, thus making transferrin saturation a less reliable laboratory index than serum ferritin under these conditions. Some investigators reported measuring serum ferritin in assessment of iron nutrition in 238 infants on seven occasions in the first year of life. The values of iron-supplemented infants remained consistently higher.

437. The answer is A (1, 2, 3). *(Oski, ed 3. pp 112–182.)* Spherocytosis can be seen in hereditary spherocytosis, G-6-PD deficiency, or ABO incompatibility. Hyperbilirubinemia has been associated with black preterm infants with G-6-PD deficiency but not with black term infants. The blood smear of the affected infant usually reveals nucleated red cells, spherocytes, poikilocytes, "blister" cells, and fragmented cells. Neonatal hyperbilirubinemia occurs in about 50 percent of patients with hereditary spherocytosis. Spherocytosis occurs in ABO incompatibility but not in Rh incompatibility. The hemolytic manifestations of ABO incompatibility and hereditary spherocytosis are very similar. One should determine the blood types of the mother and of the infant, the results of a direct Coombs' test on the infant, and the presence or absence of a family history of hemolytic disease (spherocytosis).

438–442. The answers are: 438-C, 439-E, 440-D, 441-A, 442-B. *(Nathan ed 2. pp 277, 296, 396–404, 492–502, 731–734.)* Howell-Jolly bodies (slide C) are small, spherical nuclear remnants seen in the reticulocytes and, rarely, erythrocytes of individuals who have no spleen—either owing to congenital asplenia or splenectomy—or who have a poorly functioning spleen (e.g., hyposplenism associated with sickle cell disease). Ultrafiltration of blood is a unique function of the spleen that cannot be assumed by other reticuloendothelial organs.

Basophilic stippling (slide E) represents abnormal aggregates of ribosomes within reticulocytes. This condition occurs whenever the utilization of iron for hemoglobin synthesis is impeded, as in lead intoxication and thalassemia. The presented peripheral blood smear of a child who has lead poisoning also provides evidence (microcytic, hypochromic red blood cells) of associated iron deficiency.

A target cell is an erythrocyte with a membrane that is too large for its hemoglobin content; a thin rim of hemoglobin at the cell's periphery and a small disc in the center give the cell a targetlike appearance. Target cells, which are more resistant to osmotic fragility than are other erythrocytes, are seen in children who have beta-thalassemia, hemoglobin C disease, or liver disease (e.g., obstructive jaundice or cirrhosis). Thalassemia major (slide D) can be diagnosed by the presence of poorly hemoglobinized normoblasts in addition to target cells in the peripheral blood.

Uniformly small microspherocytes (less than 6 μ in diameter) are typical of hereditary spherocytosis (slide A). Because of a decreased surface-to-volume ratio, these osmotically fragile red blood cells have an increased density of hemoglobin. Although spherical red blood cells also may appear in other hemolytic states, such as immune hemolytic anemia, microangiopathy, ABO incompatibility, and hypersplenism, their cellular volume is only irregularly augmented.

Although hemoglobin C disease (slide B) is a mild disorder, target cells constitute a far greater percentage of total red blood cells than in thalassemia major. Target cells are the only manifestations of hemoglobin C disease; targeting is so striking because hemoglobin C has a greater tendency than normal hemoglobin to aggregate and precipitate during the drying of cells on a glass slide.

443–445. The answers are: 443-D, 444-E, 445-B. *(Nathan, ed 2. pp 979–984.)* The differentiation of the types of leukemia is based mainly on morphologic characteristics as revealed by Wright's-stained smears of peripheral blood and bone marrow. Only occasionally are special cytochemical stains helpful in confirming the diagnosis.

Acute lymphoblastic leukemia is the most common type of childhood leukemia and is associated with the best prognosis. The marrow is filled with one kind of cell; most of the volume of this cell is occupied by an immature nucleus, which includes chromatin clumped around a few nucleoli. There may be folding of the nucleus. The scanty cytoplasm is blue and nongranular. Periodic acid-Schiff stain may be positive.

Acute myeloblastic leukemia is less common and has a poorer prognosis. The myeloblasts are mostly in one phase of maturity and show thin, spongy nuclear chromatin and several distinct punched-out nucleoli. The blue-gray cytoplasm is more abundant than in lymphoblasts and often contains typical Auer rods, which are abnormal lysosomes never seen in lymphoblasts. Myeloperoxidase stain may be positive.

Chronic granulocytic leukemia progresses through two stages: chronic and blastic. Bone marrow examination during the chronic phase reveals a proliferation of granulocytic cells of intermediate maturity; increased platelets also may be noted. The blastic phase, which is much harder to treat, is characterized by an increased number of less differentiated blast cells.

446–450. The answers are: 446-C, 447-E, 448-D, 449-A, 450-B. *(Altman, ed 2. pp 59–95.)* Because experimental data concerning the use of chemotherapeutic agents are incomplete and at times, perhaps, inaccurate, much of cancer chemotherapy still is given on an empirical basis. However, since the introduction of tritiated thymidine, accurate studies of DNA synthetic activities and of the proliferative characteristics of normal and leukemic cells now are possible, and a reasonably good correlation between in vivo and in vitro studies of leukemic cells has emerged. Several treatment advances, such as multimodal therapy using cytosine arabinoside in the treatment of children who have acute myelogenous leukemia, have resulted from these more sophisticated scientific studies.

The five antineoplastic drugs listed in the question all have different mechanisms of action. **Methotrexate** is a folic acid analogue that binds in a "pseudoreversible" reaction with the enzyme dehydrofolate reductase, which is essential for the synthesis of pyrimidines. **Cytosine arabinoside** (cytarabine, ara-C) is a pyrimidine analogue that impairs DNA synthesis by competitive inhibition of DNA polymerase. Both of these agents exert their antimetabolic effects during the S phase of the mitotic cycle.

Cyclophosphamide is a nitrogen mustard alkylating agent that inhibits DNA synthesis by the alkylation of purine basis. It blocks the mitotic cycle at the premitotic (G_2) stage. **Vincristine** is a vinca alkaloid, derived from the periwinkle plant; by damaging the microtubules necessary for the formation of mitotic spindles, this chemotherapeutic agent arrests mitosis during metaphase. The purine analogue **6-mercaptopurine** is an effective antineoplastic drug because it blocks purine synthesis by inhibiting two enzymatic reactions: the conversion of 5-phosphoribosyl-1-pyrophosphate to 5-phosphoribosyl-1-amine and the conversion of inosinic acid to xanthylic acid.

Endocrine, Metabolic, and Genetic Disorders

DIRECTIONS: Each question below contains five suggested responses. Select the **one best** response to each question.

451. Individuals who have a 48,XXXY karyotype are tall, mentally retarded phenotypic males having a small phallus and small, abnormal testes. Cells obtained by buccal smear would be expected to contain how many Barr bodies?

(A) One
—(B) Two
(C) Three
(D) Four
(E) None

452. All the following statements about neonatal thyrotoxicosis are true EXCEPT that

(A) it occurs equally in male and female infants
(B) it is thought to be caused by crossplacental passage of maternal thyroid-stimulating immunoglobulins (TSI)
(C) it is usually a self-limited disorder
(D) it could be life threatening and may require prompt, vigorous treatment
—(E) it does not occur when the mother is being treated with antithyroid drugs

453. True sexual precocity in girls is most likely to be caused by

(A) a feminizing ovarian tumor
(B) a gonadotropin-producing tumor
(C) a lesion of the central nervous system
(D) exogenous estrogens
—(E) early onset of "normal" puberty (constitutional)

454. A 10-year-old obese boy is diagnosed as having Cushing's syndrome on the basis of his fat distribution, his arrested growth, and the presence of hypertension, plethora, purple striae, and osteoporosis. Which of the following disorders is most likely to be responsible for the clinical picture that this boy presents?

—(A) Bilateral adrenal hyperplasia
(B) Adrenal adenoma
(C) Adrenal carcinoma
(D) Craniopharyngioma
(E) Ectopic adrenocorticotropin-producing tumor

455. According to Greek mythology, Hermaphroditus was the son of Hermes and Aphrodite. As a youth, he rejected the love of Salmacis, a river nymph. The gods granted both her wish to remain with him always and his wish to die rather than submit to her love by fusing them into one ambisexual being as they drowned in a river. All the following statements about true hermaphrodites are true EXCEPT that

(A) most are chromatin-positive
— (B) most have parents with sex-chromosome aberrations
(C) their sex-chromosome patterns may be XX, XY, or a mosaic
(D) their internal genitalia reflect the composition of their gonads
(E) they may have both a testis and an ovary

456. In many parts of the world mass screening for congenital hypothyroidism is done routinely. All the following statements are true for this disorder EXCEPT that

(A) thyroxine-binding globulin (TBG) level is usually normal
(B) serum thyroxine (T_4) level is low
— (C) clinical features of cretinism are usually apparent during the first weeks of life   2 ᵗʰ w
(D) T_3 resin uptake is low
(E) Thyroid-stimulating hormone levels (TSH) may be high, normal, or low

457. A 12-year-old girl has a mass in her neck. Physical examination reveals a thyroid nodule, but the rest of the gland is not palpable. A technetium scan reveals a "cold" nodule. The child appears to be euthyroid. Which of the following diagnoses is the LEAST likely?

(A) Simple adenoma
(B) Follicular carcinoma
(C) Papillary carcinoma
(D) A cyst
— (E) Dysgenetic thyroid gland

458. Regarding congenital adrenal hyperplasia (adrenogenital syndrome) caused by a deficiency of 21-hydroxylase, all the following statements are true EXCEPT that

(A) female infants may be virilized
(B) skin hyperpigmentation may be present
(C) infants may present with hyponatremia and hyperkalemia
— (D) male infants may have ambiguous genitalia
(E) it is an autosomal recessive disorder

459. Patients with pseudohypoparathyroidism are expected to have all the following features EXCEPT

(A) hypocalcemia
(B) hyperphosphatemia
(C) elevated concentrations of parathyroid hormone
(D) shortness of stature
— (E) rise in urinary phosphate excretion in response to the infusion of parathyroid hormone

460. Glycosylated hemoglobin (hemoglobin A1C) is often used as an indicator of control in patients with diabetes mellitus. Its level usually reflects the blood concentration of glucose over the preceding

(A) 8 hours
(B) 1 week
(C) 1 month
(D) 2 months
(E) 4 months

461. A 6-year-old girl has been referred to an endocrinologist because a reducing substance was found in her urine during a routine examination. Physical examination and glucose tolerance test results are normal; her urine reacts with Clinitest tablets but not with Clinistix. The most likely diagnosis is

(A) diabetes mellitus
(B) renal glycosuria
(C) hereditary fructose intolerance
(D) essential fructosuria
(E) deficiency of fructose-1,6-diphosphatase activity

462. A 7-day-old boy is admitted to a hospital for evaluation of vomiting and dehydration. Physical examination is otherwise normal except for minimal hyperpigmentation of the nipples. Serum sodium and potassium concentrations are 120 mEq/L and 9 mEq/L, respectively. The most likely diagnosis is

(A) pyloric stenosis
(B) congenital adrenal hyperplasia
(C) secondary hypothyroidism
(D) panhypopituitarism
(E) hyperaldosteronism

463. An infant is brought to a hospital because her wet diapers turn black when they are exposed to air. Physical examination is normal. Urine is positive both for reducing substance and when tested with ferric chloride. This disorder is caused by a deficiency of

(A) homogentisic acid oxidase
(B) phenylalanine hydroxylase
(C) L-histidine ammonia-lyase
(D) ketoacid decarboxylase
(E) isovaleryl-CoA dehydrogenase

464. Which of the following laboratory findings is unusual in patients with simple (nutritional) rickets?

(A) Aminoaciduria
(B) Hyperphosphaturia
(C) Elevated serum alkaline phosphatase levels
(D) Hypercalciuria
(E) Hypophosphatemia

465. Mental retardation of varying severity may be associated with tall stature in all the syndromes listed below EXCEPT

(A) cerebral gigantism (Sotos' syndrome)
(B) homocystinuria
(C) XXY (Kleinfelter's syndrome)
(D) Marfan's syndrome
(E) XYY

466. Hirsutism in a phenotypic female may be caused by any of the following disorders EXCEPT

(A) congenital adrenal hyperplasia (adrenogenital syndrome)
(B) Cushing's syndrome
(C) androgen-producing ovarian tumor
(D) testicular feminization—phenotypic female with intraabdominal testes and 46,XY karyotype
(E) administration of exogenous androgens

467. Maple syrup urine disease (classical branched-chain ketoaciduria) is a hereditary disorder transmitted as an autosomal recessive trait. If the gene frequency for heterozygosity is 1 in 250, the expected incidence of the disease would be

(A) 1 in 1000
(B) 1 in 25,000
(C) 1 in 62,500
(D) 1 in 250,000
(E) 1 in 625,000

468. Neonatal hypoglycemia is common in premature and small-for-gestational-age infants. The most common cause of hypoglycemia in these infants is

(A) inadequate stores of nutrients
(B) adrenal immaturity
(C) pituitary immaturity
(D) insulin excess
(E) glucagon deficiency

469. All the following statements about Wilson's disease are true EXCEPT that

(A) it is inherited as a sex-linked trait
(B) in children, it may present with hepatomegaly and liver failure
(C) ceruloplasmin levels are typically decreased
(D) total serum copper concentration is usually low
(E) it is often associated with renal disease (Fanconi syndrome)

470. A 1-day-old infant develops tetany and convulsions. Serum calcium is 6.2 mg per 100 ml. Which of the following diagnoses is the LEAST likely in this infant?

(A) Perinatal asphyxia
(B) High phosphorus intake
(C) Maternal diabetes mellitus
(D) Maternal hyperparathyroidism
(E) Prematurity

DIRECTIONS: Each question below contains four suggested responses of which **one or more** is correct. Select

A	if	**1, 2, and 3**	are correct
B	if	**1 and 3**	are correct
C	if	**2 and 4**	are correct
D	if	**4**	is correct
E	if	**1, 2, 3, and 4**	are correct

471. The adolescent athlete might appropriately be advised to increase muscle mass by

(1) taking extra vitamins
(2) doubling protein intake
(3) using hormones
(4) increasing muscle work

472. Juxtaglomerular hyperplasia (Bartter's syndrome) is characterized by which of the following conditions?

(1) Hypokalemia
(2) Hyperaldosteronism
(3) Hyperreninemia
(4) Hypertension

473. Cholecalciferol (vitamin D_3) is absorbed by the gut. In its enzymatic conversion to the active form of the vitamin, it must undergo

(1) hydroxylation at carbon 25
(2) hydroxylation at carbon 24
(3) hydroxylation at carbon 1
(4) hydroxylation at carbon 3

474. Patients with the syndrome of testicular feminization are correctly described by which of the following statements?

(1) They are genotypic females
(2) Their breasts develop at puberty
(3) Their menses can be normal
(4) They exhibit end-organ resistance to testosterone

475. Hirsutism in females may be caused by

(1) increased ovarian androgens
(2) genetic predisposition
(3) increased adrenal androgens
(4) increased testicular (ectopic) androgens

476. Known causes of primary or secondary amenorrhea include

(1) hyperprolactinemia
(2) hypothyroidism
(3) hypogonadotropic hypogonadism
(4) hyperthyroidism

477. Ketonuria usually accompanies fasting in normal children. Other true statements regarding fasting in children include which of the following?

(1) Lipolysis is enhanced
(2) Blood glucose concentration frequently decreases during 24 hours of fasting
(3) Serum fatty acid levels are high
(4) Hyperinsulinemia is present

478. Tall stature can be a feature of which of the following conditions?

(1) Familial tall stature
(2) Congenital adrenal hyperplasia (prepubertally)
(3) Marfan's syndrome
(4) Homocystinuria

479. Known causes of hyperlactaci-demia include which of the following?

(1) Pyruvate carboxylase deficiency
(2) Pyruvate dehydrogenase deficiency
(3) Fructose-1,6-diphosphatase deficiency
(4) Phosphofructokinase deficiency

480. An infant girl who has a 46,XX karyotype is hospitalized to determine the cause of her ambiguous genitalia. This child's virilization is likely to be caused by

(1) maternal exposure to progestins
(2) maternal androgen intake
(3) congenital adrenal hyperplasia
(4) neonatal Cushing's syndrome

481. Goitrous hypothyroidism can be present in a newborn infant as the result of which of the following factors?

(1) Peroxidase deficiency
(2) Maternal ingestion of thyroid hormone *e qua nhau*
(3) Maternal ingestion of iodide
(4) Thyroid-stimulating hormone deficiency — *e gây go to.*
    nsg. u thế hypothyroid e

482. A 6-year-old boy with a 2-week history of polyuria, polydipsia, and anorexia is admitted to a hospital. Likely diagnoses include which of the following?

(1) Insulin-dependent diabetes mellitus
(2) Nephrogenic diabetes insipidus *đay ra* *làm sau*
(3) Central diabetes insipidus *Sản xuất* *như sup*
(4) Phosphate diabetes

483. "Normal" or "physiological" saline has which of the following characteristics?

(1) Na^+ 154 mEq/L and Cl^- 154 mEq/L
(2) 9 g sodium chloride in 1 L of water
(3) Approximate isotonicity with blood
(4) Physiological ratio of Na^+ to Cl^-

DIRECTIONS: Each group of questions below consists of lettered headings followed by a set of numbered items. For each numbered item select the **one** lettered heading with which it is **most** closely associated. Each lettered heading may be used **once, more than once, or not at all.**

Questions 484–488

For each of the disorders listed below, select the serum concentration of calcium (Ca) and phosphate (PO$_4$) with which it is most likely to be associated.

(A) Low PO$_4$, normal Ca
(B) Low PO$_4$, high Ca
(C) Normal PO$_4$, low Ca
(D) Normal PO$_4$, normal Ca
(E) High PO$_4$, low Ca

484. Vitamin D-resistant rickets

485. Pseudohypoparathyroidism

486. Osteogenesis imperfecta

487. Hyperparathyroidism

488. Medullary thyroid carcinoma with hypercalcitoninemia

Questions 489–494

All the syndromes listed below are associated with obesity in children. For each of the other clinical findings that follow, select the syndrome with which it is most likely to be associated.

(A) Prader-Willi syndrome
(B) Laurence-Moon-Biedl syndrome
(C) Cushing's syndrome
(D) Froehlich's syndrome
(E) Pseudohypoparathyroidism

489. Cataracts

490. Hypotonia

491. Polydactyly

492. Brachydactyly

493. Basal ganglia calcification

494. Retinitis pigmentosa

Questions 495–500

For each of the following disorders, select the serum concentrations (mEq/L) of sodium (Na^+) and potassium (K^+) with which it is most likely to be associated in a dehydrated patient.

(A) Na^+ 118, K^+ 7.5
(B) Na^+ 120, K^+ 3.0
(C) Na^+ 134, K^+ 6.0
(D) Na^+ 144, K^+ 2.9
(E) Na^+ 155, K^+ 5.5

495. Salt-losing 21-hydroxylase deficiency (adrenogenital syndrome)

496. Central diabetes insipidus

497. Nephrogenic diabetes insipidus

498. Hyperaldosteronism

499. Addison's disease (in crisis)

500. Glucose-6-phosphatase deficiency (von Gierke's disease)

Endocrine, Metabolic, and Genetic Disorders

Answers

451. The answer is B. *(Behrman, ed 12. pp 306–307. Rudolph, ed 17. pp 1553–1554.)* A Barr (chromatin) body represents a partially inactivated X chromosome. The maximum number of Barr bodies in each cell nucleus is equal to the number of X chromosomes minus one. Thus, normal males (XY) and females who have Turner's syndrome (XO) tend to have no Barr bodies; normal females (XX) and males with Klinefelter's syndrome (XXY) have up to one Barr body in each cell.

452. The answer is E. *(Rudolph, ed 17. p 1535.)* Infants born to thyrotoxic mothers may be hypothyroid, euthyroid, or hyperthyroid. Neonatal thyrotoxicosis usually disappears within 2 to 4 months as the concentration of thyroid-stimulating immunoglobulins (7S gammaglobulin) diminishes. Unlike TSI, thyroid-stimulating hormone (TSH) does not cross the placenta. All forms of thyrotoxicosis are more common in females with the exception of neonatal thyrotoxicosis, which has an equal sex distribution. In severely affected infants, the disease could be fatal if not treated vigorously and promptly. Depending on the severity of the disorder, treatment with antithyroid drugs, propanolol, and digitalis may be required.

453. The answer is E. *(Behrman, ed 12. pp 1443–1445. Hung, pp 78–81.)* The term "true sexual precocity" implies that gonads have matured in response to the secretion of pituitary gonadotropins and have begun secreting sex steroids, causing the development of secondary sexual characteristics. Thus, ovarian tumors and exogenous estrogens, which suppress the function of the pituitary gland, do not cause true precocious puberty. In girls, the most common form of true precocious puberty is idiopathic and is thought to be caused by early maturation of an otherwise normal hypothalamic-pituitary-gonadal feedback system. In boys, true precocious puberty is relatively rare and is more likely to be caused by lesions of the central nervous system. Gonadotropin-producing tumors, which are very rare, may cause true precocious puberty in both sexes.

454. The answer is A. *(Behrman, ed 12. pp 1488–1489. Hung, pp 232–233.)* Although the administration of exogenous adrenocorticotropic hormone or of glucocorticoids is the most common cause of Cushing's syndrome, it may also be caused by bilateral adrenal hyperplasia. In the latter case the concentration of adrenocorti-

206

cotropic hormone may be normal or high. The basic abnormality, however, is thought to be in the hypothalamic-pituitary axis, not the adrenal gland, because a distinct pituitary adenoma is found in some patients. Furthermore, many patients who have undergone bilateral adrenalectomy develop Nelson's syndrome (invasive pituitary adenoma) despite receiving adequate cortisol replacement.

455. The answer is B. *(Behrman, ed 12. pp 1511–1512. Hung, p 340.)* True hermaphrodites by definition have both ovarian and testicular tissue. Although most are XX (chromatin-positive), some are XY, and others have chromosomal mosaicism. Although their external genitalia are ambiguous, the majority of reported hermaphroditic children have been raised as males. Ductal differentiation (development of the epididymis and vas deferens or of the fallopian tubes) is dependent on the ipsilateral presence or absence of testicular tissue, which is capable of producing androgens and müllerian inhibiting factor. Uteri are usually present. Although a familial, autosomal recessive form of true hermaphroditism has been reported, the disorder usually appears sporadically; parental sex-chromosome aberrations have no known role in its pathogenesis.

456. The answer is C. *(Rudolph, ed 17. pp 1523–1528.)* Congenital hypothyroidism may be caused by an abnormality in the thyroid gland itself (primary), in the pituitary gland (secondary), or at the level of the hypothalamus (tertiary). Thus, such a newborn is expected to have low levels of T_4 and T_3 resin uptake but, depending on the site of the defect, may have low, normal, or high concentrations of TSH. The abnormalities of thyroxine-binding globulin would give rise to abnormal thyroid function tests but not to hypothyroidism. Newborns with congenital hypothyroidism are often clinically normal at birth and diagnosis has often been delayed for several months. Mass screening has been employed to diagnose these patients within a few weeks of life before clinical signs and symptoms become manifest in order to prevent damage to the central nervous system and mental retardation.

457. The answer is E. *(Behrman, ed 12. p 1465. Hung, pp 150–155.)* A "cold" thyroid nodule may be a benign or malignant lesion; and with the exception of anaplastic carcinomas, most thyroid malignancies are slow-growing. The management of individuals who have a "cold" nodule is controversial. A common approach is to attempt to suppress the nodule with a short course of thyroid hormone administration. If the nodule persists after 3 to 6 months, surgical excision is performed. A dysgenetic thyroid gland may appear as a neck mass; as a rule, however, it is functional and thus does not appear as a "cold" nodule on thyroid scan.

458. The answer is D. *(Finberg, pp 178–179. Rudolph, ed 17. pp 1488–1491.)* 21-Hydroxylase deficiency is the most common form of congenital adrenal hyperplasia. These patients may have an impairment of the synthesis of both cortisol and aldosterone (salt-losing form) or of cortisol alone. Infants with the severe form of the disease may present with a chemical finding of hypoaldosteronism (hyponatremia and hyperkalemia). Decreased concentrations of cortisol in these patients lead to high levels of ACTH and thus hyperpigmentation of the skin and increased synthesis of adrenal androgens. Thus, female infants with 21-hydroxylase deficiency may be virilized (female pseudohermaphroditism) but males have normal external genitalia.

459. The answer is E. *(Behrman, ed 12. pp 1472–1473.)* Patients with pseudo-hypoparathyroidism have the chemical findings of hypoparathyroidism (low calcium, high phosphorus), but parathyroid hormone levels are high, indicating resistance to the action of this hormone. Thus, parathyroid hormone infusion does not produce a phosphaturic response. Phenotypically, these patients have mental retardation, shortness of stature, and obesity.

460. The answer is D. *(Behrman, ed 12. p 1414. Hung, p 385.)* Glucose is nonenzymatically attached to hemoglobin to form glycosylated hemoglobin. The major component of this reaction proceeds very slowly and is irreversible until the hemoglobin is destroyed. The concentration of glycosylated hemoglobin thus reflects glucose concentration over the half-life of the red cell, or about 2 months. Two other hemoglobins (hemoglobin A1A and A1B) have similar properties and are often measured with hemoglobin A1C.

461. The answer is D. *(Senior, Clin Perinatology 3:79, 1976. Stanbury, ed 5. pp 123–124.)* Clinitest tablets react with all reducing substances whereas Clinistix (glucose oxidase) is specific for glucose. A positive reaction with the former and a negative reaction with the latter suggest the presence of a reducing substance other than glucose in the urine. Children who have hereditary fructose intolerance as well as those who have essential fructosuria have reducing substances in their urine. Fructose intolerance, which presents during infancy, causes vomiting, hypoglycemia, and jaundice. Essential (benign) fructosuria (absence of fructokinase) is a rare autosomal recessive disorder that causes no symptoms and requires no therapy.

462. The answer is B. *(Finberg, pp 178–179. Hung, p 217. Rudolph, ed 17. pp 1488–1491.)* Salt-losing congenital adrenal hyperplasia (adrenogenital syndrome; 21-hydroxylase deficiency) usually manifests during the first 7 to 10 days of life as anorexia, vomiting, diarrhea, and dehydration. Hypoglycemia also may occur. Affected infants may have increased pigmentation, and female infants show evidence of virilization—that is, ambiguous external genitalia. Hyponatremia, hyperkalemia, and urinary sodium wasting are the usual laboratory findings. Death may occur if the diagnosis is missed and appropriate treatment is not instituted. Although adrenal aplasia, an extremely rare disorder, presents a similar clinical picture, it has an earlier onset than adrenal hyperplasia, and virilization does not occur.

463. The answer is A. *(Rudolph, ed 17. p 263.)* The infant described in the question has alkaptonuria, an autosomal recessive disorder caused by a deficiency of homogentisic acid oxidase. The diagnosis is made in infants when their urine turns black on exposure to air owing to the oxidation of homogentisic acid. Affected individuals are asymptomatic in childhood. In adults, ochronosis—the deposition of a bluish pigment in cartilage and fibrous tissue—develops; symptoms of arthritis may appear later. No specific treatment is available for individuals who have alkaptonuria. The other deficiencies listed in the question are found in phenylketonuria, histidinemia, maple syrup urine disease, and isovaleric acidemia, respectively.

464. The answer is D. *(Behrman, ed 12. p 180.)* Nutritional rickets is caused by a dietary deficiency of vitamin D and lack of exposure to sunlight. Intestinal absorption of calcium and phosphorus is diminished in vitamin D deficiency. Transient hypocalcemia stimulates the secretion of parathormone and the mobilization of calcium and phosphorus from bone; enhanced parathormone activity leads to phosphaturia and diminished excretion of calcium. In children with nutritional rickets, serum calcium concentration usually is normal and the phosphate level low. Aminoaciduria and increased serum alkaline phosphatase activity are common findings. The excretion of calcium in the urine is increased only after therapy with vitamin D has been instituted.

465. The answer is D. *(Smith, ed 3. pp 62, 64, 122, 350, 354.)* Marfan's syndrome is a genetic disorder transmitted as an autosomal dominant trait with variable expression. Individuals with this disorder usually have tall stature, arachnodactyly, subluxation of the lens, dilatation of the aorta, and dissecting aneurysm. Mental retardation is not a part of this syndrome. Vascular complications are the usual cause of death. Patients with any of the other syndromes listed have tall stature and varying degrees of mental retardation among their clinical findings.

466. The answer is D. *(Behrman, ed 12. p 1510.)* Patients with testicular feminization are genotypic males with normal testes. Complete resistance to androgens causes failure of masculinization of the external genitalia, which remain female. At puberty these individuals develop normal female breasts and body habitus despite the presence of testes and high concentrations of testosterone. Because of resistance to androgens, these patients have scant secondary sexual hair and thus do not develop hirsutism. The other disorders listed represent syndromes of excess androgens and, therefore, may cause hirsutism.

467. The answer is D. *(Rudolph, ed 17. pp 233, 251, 264.)* Maple syrup urine disease (classical branched-chain ketoaciduria) is an autosomal recessive disorder of amino acid metabolism in which the oxidative decarboxylation of branched-chain ketoacids is blocked. Because urine odor and body odor of affected individuals resemble the smell of maple syrup, the diagnosis may be suspected. The gene frequency of this disorder is approximately 1 in 250; thus, the likelihood of a union between two heterozygotes is 1 in 62,500. Because this disorder is inherited as a recessive trait, there is a 1 in 4 chance of heterozygous parents producing a homozygous offspring. Thus, the expected incidence of the disease is 1 in 250,000.

468. The answer is A. *(Cornblath, ed 2. p 191.)* Glycogen and fat stores are diminished in premature and small-for-gestational-age infants. Energy stores are inadequate to meet the energy demands after the maternal supply of glucose is interrupted at birth, and hypoglycemia ensues. Deficiency of cortisol or growth hormone is a rare cause of neonatal hypoglycemia. Insulin excess, common in infants of diabetic mothers, is unusual in other infants. Hypoglycemia associated with a deficiency of glucagon has not been well documented.

469. The answer is A. *(Rudolph, ed 17. pp 348–350. Stanbury, ed 5. pp 1255–1260.)* Wilson's disease is an autosomal recessive disorder characterized by liver disease, neurological and behavioral disturbances, renal tubular dysfunction, and eye findings. Its multisystem manifestations are caused by the deposition of copper in various tissues and therapy is aimed at the prevention of copper accumulation. The basic defect is still not known.

470. The answer is B. *(Behrman, ed 12. p 393. Hung, pp 188–189. Root, J Pediatr 88:1, 177, 1976.)* Hypocalcemia of newborn infants may be divided into two groups: early (during the first 72 hours of life) and late (after 72 hours). The most common type of early neonatal hypocalcemia is the so-called idiopathic hypocalcemia. Current data suggest that in this heterogeneous group transient hypoparathyroidism may be present; maternal hyperparathyroidism is a rare cause of transient neonatal hypoparathyroidism. Maternal complications, including diabetes mellitus and toxemia, and neonatal disorders, such as hypoxia, prematurity, sepsis, and neonatal parathyroid disease, also may cause early hypocalcemia. Hypomagnesemia and high phosphate intake are the most common factors associated with late hypocalcemia.

471. The answer is D(4). *(Forbes, ed 2. pp 63–64.)* Increased muscle work (along with increased calories) is the only appropriate way to increase muscle mass. Skin fold thickness measurements performed serially are a useful way to detect changes in the amount of body fat so that obesity can be avoided. Protein loading or using drugs, hormones, and vitamins will not be helpful and may be harmful.

472. The answer is A (1, 2, 3). *(Rudolph, ed 17. pp 1205–1206.)* Patients with Bartter's syndrome often present with failure to thrive, constipation, polyuria, vomiting, and weakness. The underlying defect is probably the failure of chloride reabsorption in the ascending limb of the loop of Henle. Laboratory findings include hypokalemia, metabolic alkalosis, hyperaldosteronism, and hyperreninemia. Hypertension is not a feature of Bartter's syndrome. Patients with chronic chloride depletion (for example, low chloride diets, chronic diuretic or laxative abuse, or chloride-losing diarrhea) may present with features of Bartter's syndrome. This syndrome may be inherited as an autosomal recessive disorder.

473. The answer is B (1, 3). *(DeLuca, Annu Rev Biochem 45:631, 1976. Hung, pp 185–187.)* Ergocalciferol (vitamin D_2) and cholecalciferol (vitamin D_3) are hydroxylated in hepatic mitochondria to form 25-hydroxy vitamin D. The rate of conversion is controlled by the concentration of 25-hydroxy vitamin D. A second hydroxylation takes place in the kidney, forming either the metabolically active compound 1,25-dihydroxy vitamin D or inactive 24,25-dihydroxy vitamin D. Formation of 1,25-dihydroxy vitamin D, the rate-limiting step in the metabolism of the vitamin, is enhanced by parathormone and low plasma phosphorus levels and is inhibited by high concentrations of calcium and phosphorus. The active form of vitamin D promotes calcium absorption in the small intestine and promotes calcium resorption from bone.

474. The answer is C (2, 4). *(Behrman, ed 12. p 1510. Hung, pp 284–285. Rudolph, ed 17. pp 1544–1548.)* Patients with testicular feminization, a genetic disorder transmitted as an X-linked recessive trait, are genetic males (karyotype 46,XY) with normal female external genitalia. The syndrome is caused by peripheral androgen resistance owing to an abnormality of receptors within the cytosol; as a result, androgen translocation into the nucleus, a crucial step in mediating androgen action, fails to occur. Diagnosis is made either during infancy or childhood when testicular tissue is found in a hernial sac at herniorrhaphy or after puberty when affected individuals present with primary amenorrhea. Well-developed vasa deferentia and epididymes are usually present; and although there is no uterus, rudimentary müllerian elements may be discovered. At puberty, individuals with testicular feminization undergo normal female breast development and may grow small amounts of sexual hair.

475. The answer is A (1, 2, 3). *(Braunwald, ed 11. pp 223–226.)* Most hirsute women have no demonstrable endocrine disorder. A genetic or constitutional cause is usually the basis of hairiness in women; for instance, Orientals and American Indians have scant body hair, whereas dark-haired individuals from Middle Eastern and Mediterranean countries tend to be hirsute. Development of sexual hair in females is dependent on the low concentration of androgens from the adrenal glands and ovaries. Excess androgen production by these organs is responsible for hirsutism in a minority of cases. Testicular tissue is not present in women. If it is present, the individual is, by definition, a hermaphrodite and usually presents with ambiguous genitalia.

476. The answer is E (all). *(Behrman, ed 12. pp 1442, 1520–1521.)* Hypogonadotropic hypogonadism caused by either hypothalamic or pituitary failure leads to ovarian understimulation and primary or secondary amenorrhea. Ovarian function is also influenced by other endocrine disorders. Hyperprolactinemia is a common cause of secondary amenorrhea and may also cause primary amenorrhea. Abnormalities of the thyroid gland (both hypo- and hyperthyroidism) also are among causes of the disturbances of ovarian function and amenorrhea.

477. The answer is A (1, 2, 3). *(Hung, pp 375–376. Senior, Pediatr Clin N Am 26:171, 1979.)* In the immediate postabsorptive state, glycogen stores are metabolized to meet energy requirements. In fasting, however, as the supply of glycogen diminishes, the body must gradually switch to lipid metabolism. Accordingly, insulin concentration is diminished and lipolysis and ketogenesis are enhanced. Serum free fatty acids and ketones are at high levels and are used as fuel. Glucose utilization diminishes and glucose concentration is maintained at a level commensurate with the ability of the body to use alternate fuels.

478. The answer is E (all). *(Behrman, ed 12. pp 1441–1442. Hung, p 81. Rudolph, ed 17. p 98.)* Tall stature in children usually is familial and cannot be traced to an underlying physiologic or metabolic abnormality. Causes of nonfamilial tall stature include pituitary gigantism (growth hormone excess), cerebral gigantism, Marfan's syndrome, homocystinuria, and chromosomal disorders, including karyotypes 47,XXY (Klinefelter's syndrome) and 47,XYY. Patients with congenital adrenal hyperplasia are tall as children but become short adults. Although boys rarely complain of tall stature, excessive height may pose psychosocial problems for girls. The use of estrogens to accelerate epiphyseal closure and reduce final adult height in girls has been advocated in the past. However, in view of the possible carcinogenicity of estrogens, this therapy must be used with caution.

479. The answer is A (1, 2, 3). *(Rudolph, ed 17. pp 267–268.)* Patients with hyperlactacidemia are a heterogeneous group with various inherited enzymatic defects. Biochemically, they are characterized by acidosis and elevated concentrations of lactate. A defect in the metabolism of pyruvate is often the underlying abnormality. Fasting hypoglycemia may be present. Patients with a deficiency of a gluconeogenic enzyme (pyruvate carboxylase, phosphoenolpyruvate carboxykinase, and fructose-1,6-diphosphatase) and those with a deficiency of pyruvate dehydrogenase complex may have hyperlactacidemia. Phosphofructokinase is an enzyme of the glycolytic pathyway and its deficiency will not give rise to high lactate levels.

480. The answer is A (1, 2, 3). *(Rudolph, ed 17. pp 1498–1500, 1542–1545.)* The most common cause of ambiguous genitalia in female infants is congenital adrenal hyperpalsia (21-hydroxylase deficiency). Maternal ingestion of androgens or progestins, the latter usually prescribed because of a threatened abortion, also may virilize a female fetus. True hermaphroditism, which is due to the presence of both ovarian and testicular tissue in the same individual, is a rare cause. Infants who have neonatal Cushing's syndrome present with massive obesity, plethora, and thinning of the skin but no evidence of virilization.

481. The answer is B (1, 3). *(Rudolph, ed 17. pp 1523–1526. Stanbury, ed 5. p 231.)* In the presence of a normal pituitary gland, a deficiency of thyroid hormones causes an elevation in thyroid-stimulating hormone levels and enlargement of the thyroid gland. Five familial disorders of thyroid hormone synthesis, including peroxidase deficiency, iodide transport defect, failure of iodotyrosine coupling, failure of iodotyrosine deiodinase activity, and altered thyroglobulin synthesis, cause goiter and hypothyroidism in neonates. In addition, maternal ingestion of goitrogens (e.g., iodide or antithyroid drugs), which cross the placenta, may cause neonatal hypothyroidism. Deficiency of thyroid-stimulating hormone may produce neonatal hypothyroidism but not gland enlargement. Thyroid hormone does not cross the placenta, and therefore, maternal ingestion would be neither beneficial nor harmful to a fetus.

482. The answer is B (1, 3). *(Finberg, pp 195–199. Rudolph, ed 17. p 297, 1162, 1476.)* Children with diabetes mellitus in early stages classically present with polyuria, polydipsia, and polyphagia. Later on, anorexia rather than polyphagia is a frequent complaint. Central diabetes insipidus is caused by a deficiency of vasopressin (antidiuretic hormone). Because the renal collecting tubules are impermeable to water, hypotonic urine is formed. Polyuria, thirst, polydipsia, and anorexia are characteristic. Children with nephrogenic diabetes insipidus have similar findings but become symptomatic shortly after birth. Phosphate diabetes (hypophosphatemic rickets) presents with the characteristic signs and symptoms of rickets and not with polyuria and polydipsia.

483. The answer is A (1, 2, 3). *(Finberg, p 237.)* "Normal" saline has an NaCl concentration of 0.9 percent (9 g/L or 154 mEq/L). This makes it isotonic with blood and body fluids so that it will not cause osmotic hemolysis or damage to tissues as solutions of lower or higher osmolality might do, which makes it useful for flushing vascular catheters. The ratio of Na^+ to Cl^- is not physiological since that ratio in blood is 140 to 100.

484–488. The answers are: 484-A, 485-E, 486-D, 487-B, 488-D. *(Behrman, ed 12. pp 1468, 1472–1475, 1645–1647, 1656.)* Vitamin D-resistant rickets is caused by a genetic abnormality in the renal tubular reabsorption of phosphate with resultant hyperphosphaturia and hypophosphatemia. No other renal tubular abnormality is present. The intestinal absorption of phosphate is also abnormal and calcium absorption from the gut may be secondarily affected. Calcium concentration is usually normal. The disorder is usually transmitted as an X-linked dominant trait.

Patients with pseudohypoparathyroidism have the same chemical abnormality (low Ca, high PO₄) as those with hypoparathyroidism. They are distinguished from the latter group by their phenotypic features and high serum concentration of para-thormone. The basic abnormality in these patients is the unresponsiveness of the renal tubules to parathyroid hormone. They are classified into two groups depending on the site of the defect. Type I patients have failure to generate cyclic AMP and do not have an increase in urinary concentration of cyclic AMP or phosphate in response to parathyroid hormone. Type II patients have a defect in the renal tubules which causes failure to respond to high concentrations of cyclic AMP. These patients, if given parathyroid hormone, have increased urinary excretion of cyclic AMP but not of phosphate.

Osteogenesis imperfecta is transmitted as an autosomal recessive (severe form) or, more commonly, autosomal dominant (mild form) disorder. The basic defect is an abnormality in the production and composition of the matrix of bone. Serum calcium and phosphate concentrations are normal.

Hyperparathyroidism is rare in children. In response to high concentrations of parathyroid hormone there is increased bone resorption. In the kidney there is in-creased excretion of phosphate and enhanced formation of 1,25-dihydroxy vitamin D. Increased formation of 1,25-dihydroxy vitamin D in turn enhances the absorption of calcium and, secondarily, of phosphorus from the gut. The net effect is hyper-calcemia and hypophosphatemia.

Medullary carcinoma of thyroid arises from the C cells of the thyroid. These tumors secrete excessive amounts of calcitonin and accordingly the concentration of this hormone in the blood is increased. Despite elevated levels of calcitonin, the serum concentration of calcium and of phosphorus is usually normal unless the patient has associated hyperparathyroidism (multiple endocrine adenomatosis, type II).

489–494. The answers are: 489-E, 490-A, 491-B, 492-E, 493-E, 494-B. *(Ru-dolph, ed 17. pp 191, 381, 1498–1501, 1568. Smith, ed 3. pp 152, 324, 442. Wilkins, ed 3. p 262.)* The Prader-Willi syndrome is a disorder consisting of hy-potonia, hypogonadism, hyperphagia, and varying degrees of mental retardation. Children affected by this syndrome exhibit little movement in utero and are hypotonic during the neonatal period. Feeding difficulties and failure to thrive may be the presenting complaints in the first year; later, obesity becomes the most common presenting complaint. The enormous food intake of affected children is thought to be due to a defect in the satiety center in the hypothalamus. Stringent caloric re-striction is the only known treatment.

Laurence-Moon-Biedl syndrome is transmitted as an autosomal recessive trait. Obesity, mental retardation, hypogonadism, polydactyly, and retinitis pigmentosa with night blindness are the principal findings in affected children. There is no known effective treatment.

The initial complaint in Cushing's syndrome may be obesity. Accumulation of fat in the face, neck, and trunk causes the characteristic ''buffalo hump'' and ''moon'' facies. Characteristic features include growth failure, muscle wasting, thinning of the skin, plethora, and hypertension. The bone age of affected patients is retarded, and osteoporosis may be present. The disorder results from an excess of glucocorticoids that may be caused by a primary adrenal abnormality (adenoma or carcinoma) or secondary hypercortisolism, which may be due to excess adrenocorticotropin. Exogenous glucocorticoids administered in supraphysiologic doses for a prolonged period of time will produce a similar picture in normal subjects.

Pseudohypoparathyroidism is a familial disorder transmitted as an X-linked trait. Affected patients have biochemical findings (low serum calcium and high serum phosphorus levels) similar to those associated with hypoparathyroidism, but they also have high levels of endogenous parathormone; in addition, exogenous parathormone fails to increase their phosphate excretion or raise their serum calcium level. The defect in these patients appears to be either at the hormone receptor site or in the adenylate cyclase-cyclic AMP system. The symptoms of pseudohypoparathyroidism are due to hypocalcemia. Affected children are short, round-faced, and mildly retarded. Metacarpals and metatarsals are shortened, and metastatic calcifications, basal ganglia calcifications, and cataracts may be present. The current treatment consists of large doses of vitamin D and reduction of the phosphate load.

Froehlich's syndrome was described originally in an obese boy with sexual infantilism and shortness of stature but is no longer used as a diagnostic term.

495–500. The answers are: 495-A, 496-E, 497-E, 498-D, 499-A, 500-B. *(Finberg, pp 171–183, 198–199. Hung, pp 105, 109, 110, 227, 240. Rudolph, ed 17. pp 292, 1476–1478, 1501–1502.)* In the salt-losing variety of 21-hydroxylase deficiency, the synthesis of both mineralocorticoids (e.g., aldosterone) and cortisol is impaired. Aldosterone deficiency impairs the exchange of potassium for sodium in the distal renal tubule. Affected patients have hyponatremia and hyperkalemia. Dehydration, hypotension, and shock may be present.

In the absence of vasopressin, renal collecting tubules are impermeable to water, resulting in the excretion of hypotonic urine. Patients with diabetes insipidus present with polyuria and polydipsia. Net loss of water leads to dehydration and hemoconcentration and, therefore, to relatively high serum concentrations of sodium and potassium. Patients with nephrogenic diabetes insipidus have similar laboratory findings. This genetic disorder is unresponsive to antidiuretic hormone (ADH). These patients are unable to concentrate their urine and present in the neonatal period with hypernatremic dehydration.

In hyperaldosteronism, renal tubular sodium-potassium exchange is enhanced. Hypokalemia, hypernatremia, hyperchloremia, and akalosis are the usual findings. Primary hyperaldosteronism (Conn's syndrome) is very rare in children.

Addison's disease is associated with a combined deficiency of glucocorticoids and mineralocorticoids. Resorption of sodium and excretion of potassium and hydrogen ions are impaired at the level of the distal renal tubules. Sodium loss results in loss of water and depletion of blood volume. Individuals with compensated Addison's disease may have relatively normal physical and laboratory findings; Addisonian crisis, however, characteristically produces hyponatremia, hyperkalemia, and shock. The pathophysiology of the serum electrolyte abnormalities in this disorder is the same as in the salt-losing variety of adrenogenital syndrome.

Patients with a deficiency of glucose-6-phosphatase (von Gierke's disease) are, as a rule, hyperlipemic. Increased triglyceride concentration in the serum decreases the volume of the aqueous compartment. Because electrolytes are present only in the aqueous compartment of the serum but are expressed in milliequivalents per liter of serum as a whole, the concentrations of sodium and potassium are factitiously low in these patients.

Bibliography

Adams F, Emmanouilides GC (eds): *Moss' Heart Disease in Infants, Children and Adolescents,* 3rd ed. Baltimore, Waverly Press, 1983.

Adams RG, Lyon G: *Neurology of Hereditary Metabolic Diseases of Children.* New York, McGraw-Hill, 1981.

Alpert E: Pathogenesis of arthritis associated with viral hepatitis. *N Engl J Med* 285:185–189, 1971.

Altman AJ, Schwartz AD: *Malignant Diseases of Infancy, Childhood and Adolescence,* 2nd ed. Philadelphia, WB Saunders, 1983.

American Academy of Pediatrics, American College of Obstetrics and Gynecology [AAP-ACOG]: *Guidelines for Perinatal Care,* 1983.

American Academy of Pediatrics, Committee on Accident and Poison Prevention [AAP-CAPP]: *Handbook of Common Poisonings in Children,* ed 2, ed by R Aronow, 1983.

American Academy of Pediatrics, Committee on Infectious Diseases [AAP-CID]: *Report,* ed 20, 1986.

American Academy of Pediatrics, Committee on Nutrition [AAP-CN]: Iron supplementation for infants. *Pediatrics* 58:765, 1976.

Avery GB (ed): *Neonatology: Pathophysiology and Management of the Newborn,* 2nd ed. Philadelphia, JB Lippincott, 1981.

Avery ME, Taeusch HW Jr (eds): *Schaffer's Diseases of the Newborn,* 5th ed. Philadelphia, WB Saunders, 1984.

Baraff LJ, Wilkins J, Wehrle PF: The role of antibiotics, immunization, and adenoviruses in pertussis. *Pediatrics* 61:224–230, 1978.

Behrman RE, Vaughn VC III: *Nelson Textbook of Pediatrics,* 12th ed. Philadelphia, WB Saunders, 1983.

Bell WE, McCormick WF: *Increased Intracranial Pressure in Children,* 2nd ed, vol 8. Philadelphia, WB Saunders, 1978.

Blacklow NR: Viral gastroenteritis. *N Engl J Med* 304:397–406, 1981.

Braunwald E: *Heart Disease: A Textbook of Cardiovascular Medicine,* 2nd ed. Philadelphia, WB Saunders, 1984.

Braunwald E, et al: *Harrison's Principles of Internal Medicine,* 11th ed. New York, McGraw-Hill, 1987.

Brown JK: Migraine and migraine equivalents in children. *Develop Med Child Neurol* 19:683–692, 1977.

Browne TB: Valproic acid. *N Engl J Med* 302:661–665, 1980.

Cines DB, Dusak B, Tomaski A, et al: Immune thrombocytopenia and pregnancy. *N Engl J Med* 306:826, 1982.

Cornblath M, Schwartz R: *Disorders of Carbohydrate Metabolism in Infancy*, 2nd ed. Philadelphia, WB Saunders, 1976.

Dallman PR: Iron deficiency in infancy and childhood. *Report of the International Nutritional Anemia Consultative Group (INACG)*, 1979.

DeGroot LJ, et al: *The Thyroid and Its Diseases*, 5th ed. New York, John Wiley, 1984.

Delgado-Escueta AV, et al: *Advances in Neurology*, New York, Raven Press, 1983.

De Luca HF, Schnoes HK: Metabolism and mechanism of action of vitamin D. *Annu Rev Biochem* 45:631, 1976.

DeVivo DC, Keating JP, Haymond MW: Acute encephalopathy with fatty infiltration of the viscera. *Pediatr Clin North Am* 23:527–540, 1976.

Dillon HC: Impetigo contagiosa: Suppurative and non-suppurative complications. *Am J Dis Child* 115:530–541, 1968.

Dodge PR: Myotonic dystrophy in infancy and childhood. *Pediatrics* 35:3–19, 1965.

Dodge PR, Swartz MN: Bacterial meningitis—a review of selected aspects. *N Engl J Med* 272:954–960, 1003–1010, 1965.

Dubowitz V: *Muscle Disorders in Childhood*, vol 16. Philadelphia, WB Saunders, 1978.

Faerø O, Kastrup KW, Nielson EL, et al: Successful prophylaxis of febrile convulsions with phenobarbital. *Epilepsia* 13:279–285, 1972.

Fanaroff AA, Martin RJ (eds): *Behrman's Neonatal Perinatal Medicine*, 3rd ed. St. Louis, CV Mosby, 1983.

Feder HM Jr: Occult pneumococcal bacteremia and the febrile infant and young child—clinical review. *Clin Pediatr* 19:457–462, 1980.

Fekety R: Recent advances in bacterial diarrhea. *Rev Infect Dis* 5:246–257, 1983.

Finberg L, Kravath RE, Fleischman AR: *Water and Electrolytes in Pediatrics*. Philadelphia, WB Saunders, 1982.

Fishman RA: *Cerebrospinal Fluid in Diseases of the Nervous System*. Philadelphia, WB Saunders, 1980.

Fleischer GR: Falsely normal radionucleide scans for osteomyelitis. *Am J Dis Child* 134:499–502, 1980.

Forbes GB, Woodruff CW: *Pediatric Nutrition Handbook*. American Academy of Pediatrics, Committee on Nutrition, 1985.

Gellis SS (ed): *Year Book of Pediatrics*. Chicago, Year Book Medical, 1978.

Gellis SS, Kagan BM (eds): *Current Pediatric Therapy*, 11th ed. Philadelphia, WB Saunders, 1984.

Gilman AG, et al (eds): *Goodman and Gilman's The Pharmacological Basis of Therapeutics*, 7th ed. New York, Macmillan, 1985.

Gomez M (ed): *Tuberous Sclerosis*. New York, Raven Press, 1979.

Gordon N: *Pediatric Neurology for the Clinician*. Philadelphia, JB Lippincott, 1976.

Greenberger N: Medium chain triglycerides, physiological considerations and clinical implications. *N Engl J Med* 280:1045–1058, 1969.

Greeson NT, Kirkpatrick JA, Gradang BR, et al: Gastric antral narrowing in chronic granulomatous disease of childhood. *Pediatrics* 54:456, 1974.

Guggenheim MA, et al: Progressive neuromuscular disease in children with chronic cholestasis and vitamin E deficiency: Diagnosis and treatment with alpha tocopherol. *J Pediatr* 100:51–58, 1982.

Handsfield HH, et al: Epidemiology of penicillinase-producing *Neisseria gonorrhoeae* infections. *N Engl J Med* 306:950–954, 1982.

Higby DJ: Granulocyte transfusions: Current status. *Blood* 55:2–8, 1980.

Hrachovy RA, et al: Double-blind study of ACTH vs prednisone therapy in infantile spasms. *J Pediatr* 103:641–645, 1983.

Hubbard JP: *Measuring Medical Education*, 2nd ed. Philadelphia, Lea & Febiger, 1978.

Hung W, August GP, Glasgow AM: *Pediatric Endocrinology*. New Hyde Park, N.Y., Medical Examination Publishing, 1983.

Illingworth RS: *The Development of the Infant and Young Child: Normal and Abnormal*, 8th ed. New York, Longman, 1984.

Isler W: *Clinics in Developmental Medicine*. Philadelphia, JB Lippincott, 1971.

Johnson: *N Engl J Med* 310:137–141, 1984.

Karayalcin G, Hassani N, Abrams M: Cholelithiasis in children with sickle cell disease. *Am J Dis Child* 233:306, 1979.

Keith JD, Rowe RD, Vlad P: *Heart Disease in Infancy and Childhood*, 3rd ed. New York, Macmillan, 1978.

Kelley VC: *Practice of Pediatrics*. New York, Harper & Row, 1984.

Kendig EL, Chernick V (eds): *Disorders of the Respiratory Tract in Children*, 4th ed. Philadelphia, WB Saunders, 1983.

Kerr DN, Harrison CV, Sherlock S, et al: Congenital hepatic fibrosis. *Q J Med* 30:91–117, 1961.

Kohl S: *Yersinia enterocolitica* infections in children. *Pediatr Clin North Am* 26:433–443, 1979.

Kravath RE, Pollak CP, Borowiecki B: Hypoventilation during sleep in children who have lymphoid airway obstruction treated by nasopharyngeal tube and T and A. *Pediatrics* 59:865, 1977.

Krugman S, Ward R, Katz SC: *Infectious Diseases of Children,* 7th ed. St. Louis, CV Mosby, 1980.

Levin DL, Morriss FC, Moore GC: *A Practical Guide to Pediatric Intensive Care,* 2nd ed. St. Louis, CV Mosby, 1984.

Levine, AD (ed): *Cancer in the Young.* New York, Masson Publishing USA, 1982.

Lindenbaum J: Megaloblastic anemia and neutrophil hypersegmentation. *Br J Haematol* 44:511–513, 1979.

Luban NLC, Leikin SL, August GA: Growth and development in sickle cell anemia: Preliminary report. *Am J Pediatr Hematol/Oncol* 4(1):61–65, 1982.

Lumicao GG, Heggie AD: Chlamydial infections. *Pediatr Clin North Am* 26:269–282, 1979.

Lux SE, Wolfe LC: Inherited disorders of the red cell membrane skeleton. *Pediatr Clin North Am* 27:463–486, 1980.

Mauer AM: Therapy of acute lymphoblastic leukemia in childhood. *Blood* 56:1–10, 1980.

McRae DL: Observations on craniolacunia. *Acta Radiol* (Diagn) 5:55–64, 1966.

Meissner HC: Lyme disease first observed to be aseptic meningitis. *Am J Dis Child* 136:465–467, 1982.

Meissner HC, Smith AL: The current status of chloramphenicol. *Pediatrics* 64:348–356, 1979.

Menkes JH: *Textbook of Child Neurology,* 2nd ed. Philadelphia, Lea & Febiger, 1980.

Monreal FJ: Asymmetric crying facies: An alternative interpretation. *Pediatrics* 65:146–149, 1980.

Nathan DG, Oski FA: *Hematology of Infancy and Childhood,* 2nd ed. Philadelphia, WB Saunders, 1981.

Nelson KB, Ellenberg JH: Predictors of epilepsy in children who have experienced febrile seizures. *N Engl J Med* 295:1029–1033, 1976.

Nelson KB, Eng G: Congenital hypoplasia of the depressor anguli oris muscle: Differentiation from congenital facial palsy. *J Pediatr* 81:16–20, 1972.

Neville BG: Central nervous system involvement in leukemia. *Dev Med Child Neurol* 14:75–78, 1972.

Oski FA, Naiman JL: *Hematologic Problems in the Newborn,* 3rd ed. Philadelphia, WB Saunders, 1982.

Oski FA, Stockman JA: Anemia due to inadequate iron sources or poor iron utilization. *Pediatr Clin North Am* 27:237–253, 1980.

Pape KE, Pickering D: Asymmetric crying facies: An index of other congenital anomalies. *J Pediatr* 81:21–30, 1972.

Partin JD: Mitochondrial ultra-structure in Reye's syndrome. *N Engl J Med* 285:1139–1143, 1971.

Perloff JK: *The Clinical Recognition of Congenital Heart Disease,* 2nd ed. Philadelphia, WB Saunders, 1978.

Peter G, Smith AL: Group A streptococcal infections of the skin and pharynx. *N Engl J Med* 297:311–317, 365–370, 1977.

Plum F, Posner JB: *The Diagnosis of Stupor and Coma,* 3rd ed. Philadelphia, FA Davis, 1980.

Pollack JD: *Reye's Syndrome.* New York, Grune & Stratton, 1975.

Prensky AL, Sommer D: Diagnosis and treatment of migraine in children. *Neurology* 29:506–510, 1979.

Price RA, Jamieson PA: The central nervous system in childhood leukemia. II. Subacute leucoencephalopathy. *Cancer* 35:306–318, 1975.

Prince AS, Neu HC: Antibiotic-associated pseudomembranous colitis in children. *Pediatr Clin North Am* 26:261–268, 1979.

Reye RD: Encephalopathy and fatty degeneration of the viscera: A disease entity in childhood. *Lancet* 2:749–757, 1963.

Roberts WC: *Cardiology.* New York, Yorke Medical Books, 1983.

Root AW, Harrison HE: Recent advances in calcium metabolism. *J Pediatr* 88:1–18, 177–179, 1976.

Rubenstein L, Herman MM, Long TF, et al: Disseminated necrotizing leucoencephalopathy: A complication of treated central nervous system leukemia and lymphoma. *Cancer* 35:291–305, 1975.

Rudolph AM, et al (eds): *Pediatrics,* 17th ed. New York: Appleton-Century-Crofts, 1982.

Sabesin SM, Koff RS: Pathogenesis of experimental viral hepatitis. *N Engl J Med* 290:944–950, 996–1002, 1974.

Sanford JP: Legionnaire's disease—the first thousand days. *N Engl J Med* 300:654–656, 1979.

Sato S, et al: Valproic acid versus ethosurimide in the treatment of absence seizures. *Neurology* 32:157–163, 1982.

Scarpelli EM, Auld PAM, Goldman HS (eds): *Pulmonary Disease of the Fetus, Newborn and Child.* Philadelphia, Lea & Febiger, 1978.

Schapiro RL: *Clinical Radiology of the Pediatric Abdomen Gastrointestinal Tract.* Baltimore, University Park Press, 1979.

Scharli, A, Sieber WK, Kiesewetter WB: Hypertrophic pyloric stenosis at Children's Hospital of Pittsburgh from 1912 to 1967: A critical view. *J Pediatr Surg* 4:108–114, 1969.

Schiff L: *Diseases of the Liver,* 5th ed. Philadelphia, JB Lippincott, 1982.

Senior B, Sadeghi-Nejad A: The glycogenoses and other inherited disorders of carbohydrate metabolism. *Clin Perinatol* 3:79, 1976.

Senior B, Wolfsdorf JI: Hypoglycemia in children. *Pediatr Clin North Am* 26:171–185, 1979.

Seto DSY: Viral hepatitis. *Pediatr Clin North Am* 26:305–314, 1979.

Shapiro AK, Shapiro E: Tourette syndrome: Clinical aspects, treatment, and etiology. *Semin Neurol* 2:373–385, 1982.

Silverman A, Roy CC, Cozzetto FJ: *Pediatric Clinical Gastroenterology,* 3rd ed. St. Louis, CV Mosby, 1983.

Silverman WA: *Human Experimentation: A Guided Step into the Unknown.* New York, Oxford, 1985.

Singer WD, Rabe EF, Haller JS: The effect of ACTH therapy upon infantile spasms. *J Pediatr* 96:485–489, 1980.

Sleisenger MH, Fordtran JS: *Gastrointestinal Disease: Pathophysiology, Diagnosis, Management,* 3rd ed. Philadelphia, WB Saunders, 1983.

Smith DW: *Recognizable Patterns of Human Malformation: Genetic, Embryologic and Clinical Aspects,* 3rd ed. Philadelphia, WB Saunders, 1982.

Stanbury JB, Wyngaarden JB, Fredrickson DS: The Metabolic Basis of Inherited Disease, 5th ed. New York, McGraw-Hill, 1983.

Steinhoff MC: Rotavirus: The first five years. *J Pediatr* 96:611–622, 1980.

Sullivan DW: Hereditary spherocytosis. *Pediatr Ann* 9:38–42, 1980.

Sullivan JL: Epstein-Barr virus and X-linked lymphoproliferative syndrome *Adv Pediatr* 31:365–399, 1984.

Swaiman DF, Wright FS (eds): *The Practice of Pediatric Neurology.* 2nd ed. St. Louis, CV Mosby, 1982.

Taylor-Robinson D, McCormack WM: The genital mycoplasmas. *N Engl J Med* 302:1003–1010, 1063–1067, 1980.

Thompson JA: Infant botulism: Clinical spectrum and epidemiology. *Pediatrics* 66:936–942, 180.

Thomsett MJ, et al: Endocrine and neurologic outcome in childhood craniopharyngioma: Review of effect of treatment in 42 patients. *J Pediatr* 97:728–735, 1980.

Tipple MA, Been NO, Saxon EM: Clinical characteristics of the afebrile pneumonia associated with *Chlamydia trachomatis* infection in infants less than 6 months of age. *Pediatrics* 63:192–197, 1979.

Torphy DD, Bond WW: *Campylobacter* fetus infections in children. *Pediatrics* 64:896–903, 1979.

Trier JS: Diagnostic value per oral biopsy of the proximal small intestine. *N Engl J Med* 285:1470, 1973.

Walton JN: *Disorders of Voluntary Muscle,* 4th ed. New York, Churchill Livingstone, 1981.

Welch KJ, Randolph JG, Ravitch MM, et al: *Pediatric Surgery,* 4th ed. Chicago, Year Book Medical Publishers, 1986.

Wilkins L: *The Diagnosis and Treatment of Endocrine Disorders in Childhood and Adolescence,* 3rd ed. Springfield, Charles C Thomas, 1966.

Williams WJ, et al: *Hematology,* 2nd ed. New York, McGraw-Hill, 1977.

Wilson (ed): *Williams Textbook of Endocrinology,* 7th ed. Philadelphia, WB Saunders, 1985.

Ziai, M: *Pediatrics,* 3rd ed. Boston, Little, Brown, 1984.